Managing
Gynaecological
Emergencies

Managing
Gynaecological
Emergencies

C. Cox
FRCS (Ed) FRCOG
Consultant Obstetrician and Gynaecologist,
New Cross Hospital, Wolverhampton WV10 0QP, UK

K. Grady
BSc FRCA
Consultant Anaesthetist,
South Manchester University Hospitals' NHS Trust,
Southmoor Road, Manchester M23 9LT, UK

K. Hinshaw
MB BS MRCOG
Consultant Obstetrician and Gynaecologist,
Sunderland Royal Hospital, Kayll Road,
Sunderland, Tyne and Wear SR4 7TP, UK

© BIOS Scientific Publishers Limited, 2003

First published in 2003

A CIP catalogue record for this book is available from the British Library.

ISBN 1 85996 310 2

BIOS Scientific Publishers Ltd
9 Newtec Place, Magdalen Road, Oxford OX4 1RE, UK
Tel. +44 (0)1865 726286. Fax +44 (0)1865 246823
World Wide Web home page: http: //www.bios.co.uk/

Important Note from the Publisher
The information contained within this book was obtained by BIOS Scientific Publishers Ltd from sources believed by us to be reliable. However, while every effort has been made to ensure its accuracy, no responsibility for loss or injury whatsoever occasioned to anyperson acting or refraining from action as a result of information contained herein can be accepted by the authors or publishers.

The reader should remember that medicine is a constantly evolving science and while the authors and publishers have ensured that all dosages, applications and practices are based on current indications, there may be specific practices which differ between communities. You should always follow the guidelines laid down by the manufacturers of specific products and the relevant authorities in the country in which you are practising.

Production Editor: Phil Dines
Typeset by Saxon Graphics Ltd, Derby, UK
Printed by Biddles Ltd, Guildford, UK

CONTENTS

4. EMERGENCIES IN UROGYNAECOLOGY

5. EMERGENCIES IN GYNAECOLOGICAL ONCOLOGY
S. Houghton and C. Cox

CONTRIBUTORS

Adair, S MB BCh BAO MRCOG
Specialist Registrar in Obstetrics & Gynaecology, Royal Jubilee Maternity Service, Royal Victoria Hospital, Grosvenor Road, Belfast, BT12 6BA, UK

Allenby, K MB BS DRCOG MRCOG Cert Med Ed
Consultant Obstetrician & Gynaecologist, Clinical Director Women's Health, Middlemore Hospital, Private Bag 93311, Otahuhu, Auckland, New Zealand

Cameron, H MB BS FRCOG
Consultant Obstetrician & Gynaecologist, Sunderland Royal Hospital, Kayll Road, Sunderland, Tyne & Wear, SR4 7TP, UK

Evans, D MB BS FRCOG
Consultant Obstetrician & Gynaecologist, North Tyneside General Hospital, Rake Lane, North Shields, Tyne & Wear, NE29 8NH, UK

Guirguis, M MB BCh MSc MRCOG
Locum Consultant, Guy's and St Thomas' Hospital, St Thomas' Street, London, SE1 9RT, UK

Hooper, P MB MRCOG
Consultant Obstetrician & Gynaecologist, Nottingham University Hospital Queen's Medical Centre, Nottingham NG7 2UH, UK

Houghton, SJ MB ChB MRCOG
Consultant Obstetrician & Gynaecologist, Good Hope Hospital NHS Trust, Rectory Road, Sutton Coldfield, West Midlands, B75 7RR, UK

Lieberman, I MB BS FRCA
Consultant Anaesthetist, South Manchester University Hospitals' NHS Trust, Manchester, M23 9LT, UK

Mann, CH MD MRCOG
Senior Lecturer in Obstetrics & Gynaecology, Birmingham Women's Hospital, Metchley Park Road, Edgbaston, Birmingham, B15 2TG, UK

McCabe, N MB BCh BAO MRCOG
Consultant Obstetrician & Gynaecologist, Lagan Valley Hospital, Hillsborough Road, Lisburn, County Down, BT28 1JP, UK

Miller, B MB ChB FRCA DA
Consultant Anaesthetist, Royal Bolton Hospital, Minerva Road, Farnworth, Bolton, BL4 0JR, UK,

Moran, PA MRCOG
Consultant, Worcester Royal Infirmary, Rankswood Branch, Newtown Road, Worcester, WR5 1HN, UK

Roberts, M MD MRCOG
Consultant Gynaecologist, Women's Services, Royal Victoria Infirmary, Newcastle upon Tyne, Tyne & Wear, NE1 4LP, UK

Sorinola, O MB BS MRCOG MedSc
Consultant Obstetrician & Gynaecologist, Warwick Hospital, Lakin Road, Warwick, Warwickshire, CV34 5BW, UK

Sullivan, H MD MRCOG
Consultant Obstetrician & Gynaecologist, New Cross Hospital, Wolverhampton, West Midlands, WV10 0QP, UK

Wright, JT FRCOG
Consultant in Obstetrics & Gynaecology, St Peter's Hospital, Guildford Road, Chertsey, Surrey, KT16 0PZ, UK

Wykes, CB MBBS BSc MRCOG
Specialist Registrar in Obstetrics & Gynaecology, New Cross Hospital, Wolverhampton, West Midlands, WV10 0QP, UK

Contributors

ABBREVIATIONS

ABGs	arterial blood gases
ACE	angiotensin converting enzyme
AED	automated external defibrillator
ALS	advanced life support
ANA	anti-nuclear antibody
AP	antero-posterior
APTT	activated partial thromboplastin time
ARF	acute renal failure
ASD	atrial septal defect
AXR	abdominal X-ray
BP	blood pressure
BSO	bilateral salpingo-oophorectomy
CEA	carcino-embryonic antigen
CHM	complete hydatidiform mole
CISC	clean intermittent self-catheterization
COCP	combined oral contraceptive pill
CPR	cardiopulmonary resuscitation
CPS	Crown Prosecution Service
C-RP	C-reactive protein
CT	computerised tomography
CVP	central venous pressure
CXR	chest X-ray
DES	diethylstilboestrol
DIC	disseminated intravascular coagulation
DVT	deep venous thrombosis
ECG	electrocardiogram
EP	ectopic pregnancy
EPAU/C	early pregnancy assessment unit/clinic
ERPC	evacuation of retained products of conception
EUA	examination under anaesthesia
FBC	full blood count
FFP	fresh frozen plasma
FME	forensic medical examiner
GA	general anaesthesia
G+S	group and save
GTD	gestational trophoblastic disease
GTTs	gestational trophoblastic tumours
GUM	genito-urinary medicine
hCG	human chorionic gonadotrophin
HDU	High Dependency Unit
HIV	human immunodeficiency virus
hMG	human menopausal gonadotrophin
HRT	hormone replacement therapy
HSG	hysterosalpingogram
HVS	high vaginal swab
ICU	Intensive Care Unit
IDS	interval debulking surgery
IM	intramuscular
IUCD	intrauterine contraceptive device

IUD	intrauterine death
IV	intravenous
IVP	intravenous pyelogram
IVS	intravascular space
LA	local anaesthesia
LFTs	liver function tests
LLETZ	large loop excision of the transformation zone
LMP	last menstrual period
LMW	low molecular weight
LND	lymph node dissection
MI	myocardial infarction
MODS	multiorgan dysfunction syndrome
MRI	magnetic resonance imaging
MSU	midstream specimen of urine
MTX	methotrexate
NBM	nil by mouth
NEC	necrotizing enterocolitis
NSAID	non-steroidal anti-inflammatory drug
OHSS	ovarian hyperstimulation syndrome
OI	ovulation induction
PCA	patient-controlled analgesia
PCOD	polycystic ovarian disease
PCWP	pulmonary capillary wedge pressure
PDA	patent ductus arteriosus
PE	pulmonary embolism
PEA	pulseless electrical activity
PEFR	peak expiratory flow rate
PG	prostaglandin
PHM	partial hydatidiform mole
PID	pelvic inflammatory disease
PO	orally
POC	products of conception
PONV	post-operative nausea and vomiting
POP	progesterone only pill
PR	per rectum
PRN	as necessary
PSTT	placental site trophoblastic tumour
PT	pregnancy test
PU	peptic ulceration
PV	'per vaginum' (internal vaginal examination)
RAST	radioallergosorbent testing
RR	respiratory rate
RTA	road traffic accident
RUQ	right upper quadrant
SaO2	arterial oxygen saturation
SI	sexual intercourse
SIRS	systemic inflammatory response syndrome
SPC	suprapubic catheter
SpR	Specialist Registrar
STD	sexually transmitted disease
SVR	systemic vascular resistance
TA	transabdominal
TAH	total abdominal hysterectomy

TCI	target controlled infusion
TFTs	thyroid function tests
TIVA	total intravenous anaesthesia
TSS	toxic shock syndrome
TV	transvaginal
U&E	urea and electrolytes
UTI	urinary tract infection
VAIN	vaginal intraepithelial neoplasia
VAT	vacuum aspiration termination
VE	vaginal examination
VF	ventricular fibrillation
VIN	vulval intraepithelial neoplasia
V/Q	ventilation/perfusion
VSD	ventricular septal defect
VT	ventricular tachycardia
WCC	white cell count
X Match	cross match

PREFACE

This book is written for gynaecologists in training. However, we hope that the concise format will help others, including general practice trainees and specialist nurses, in the management of gynaecological emergencies. Our aim has been to produce a single text, containing a safe and pragmatic approach to the multitude of practical problems and professional dilemmas facing the gynaecologist in day-to-day emergency practice. The book not only discusses specific gynaecological emergencies, but also reviews critical care of medical emergencies as they befall the gynaecology patient, as well as peri-operative assessment. It is written in a style designed to make access to information as easy as possible.

The book is a collection of "Action Plans" for emergency care. The management plans are concise but comprehensive. The aim is to take the reader through logical, safe steps. It may not be necessary to work through to the end of each plan: this will depend on patient condition and the effectiveness of preceding steps. It is recommended that to manage the condition comprehensively, the whole chapter is consulted in moments of less urgency.

The text is divided into sections, covering emergencies and complications in: general gynaecology, early pregnancy, gynaecological surgery, urogynaecology and gynaecological oncology. The appendices cover problems and issues arising in the peri-operative period, commoner medical emergencies affecting gynaecology inpatients and the often difficult professional issues of risk management and consent.

This is a sister book to the text *Managing Obstetric Emergencies* (BIOS, 1999).

We dedicate this book to our late friend and colleague Professor Richard Johanson, whose premature death on 21st February 2002 was a significant loss to the specialty of obstetrics and gynaecology. It was Richard's intention to act as guest editor to this text and it was his inspiration and encouragement that made it possible. We are also grateful to all of our co-authors who have given freely of their time and expertise. Finally, we must acknowledge the support of the editorial staff at BIOS who have cajoled and encouraged us over the last 18 months!

Charles Cox
Kate Grady
Kim Hinshaw

FOREWORD

Managing Gynaecological Emergencies is a practical textbook developed and produced by clinicians with extensive experience of training and education in our speciality.

The book is laid out in a useful format, which follows "Action Plans" for the management of a comprehensive range of gynaecological emergencies. This format provides an infrastructure for the rapid management of acute and sometimes life-threatening conditions. As such, this will be an invaluable tool for all those having to come to grips with gynaecological emergencies for the first time. The sections which address complications associated with surgery are especially useful and should be made available to everyone involved in post-operative patient management.

Many of the principal editors and authors have also contributed to the RCOG Distance Programme modules in StratOG. This book complements StratOG very well and will be valuable to trainees in Obstetrics and Gynaecology undertaking the StratOG programme.

The style of the book facilitates ease of use and the format is intuitive. The reader is led logically through the clinical management of each condition. Finally, the book is truly problem-orientated, thereby facilitating active learning.

Sean Duffy MD FRCS (Glasg) FRCOG
Senior Lecturer
Academic Division of Obstetrics and Gynaecology
University of Leeds
Editor in Chief RCOG StratOG

ACUTE ABDOMINAL PAIN

Niamh McCabe and Kim Hinshaw

Acute abdominal pain is one of the commonest gynaecological presentations and has a myriad of causes. Gynaecological, surgical and medical causes may need to be considered. Age is an important factor in considering the likely diagnosis. The non-gynaecological causes which should be considered here are similar to those described in the chapter on alternative causes of acute abdominal pain in early pregnancy. However, a few additional causes become relevant in the post-menopausal population. In this chapter the gynaecological causes of acute abdominal pain will be brought together and an action plan for management discussed.

ACTION PLAN

1 **If shocked, resuscitate – follow ABCs. Call for appropriate help**

2 **Review history. Women of reproductive age – consider pregnancy**

3 **Perform general examination**
- Pulse, blood pressure, temperature (but remember that young fit women will maintain a normal blood pressure in the presence of significant intra-abdominal bleeding).
- Note degree of distress.

4 **Perform abdominal examination**
- Check for the presence of scars, guarding, rebound and masses.

5 **Pelvic examination (including speculum and swabs)**

6 **Establish iv access**

7 **Analgesia**
- Opioids or NSAID depending on severity of pain and differential diagnosis.

8 **Consider gynaecological causes of acute abdominal pain**

9 **Consider non-gynaecological causes of abdominal pain (review list below)**

10 **Investigations (as dictated by clinical situation)**

Common
- FBC.
- Urine microscopy/MSU.
- Pregnancy test.
- Endocervical swabs.
- Amylase.
- U&E.

Consider
- Abdominal/pelvic USS.
- AXR/CXR.

Selective
- Group and save or X-match.
- ESR or C-reactive protein.

- LFTs.
- Faecal occult bloods.
- CA125.

11 **Consider need for laparoscopy or proceed directly to laparotomy**

CONSULT OTHER TOPICS

Childhood emergencies (p 47)
Early pregnancy emergencies – admitting patients to the ward (p 73)
Ectopic pregnancy (p 76)
Gynaecological emergencies in the older woman (p 52)
Ovarian hyperstimulation syndrome (p 10)
Scan findings relevant to the Early Pregnancy Assessment Unit (p 68)
Surgical management of ovarian cysts in the pregnant and non-pregnant (p 6)
Upper tract pelvic infection (p 13)

SUPPLEMENTARY INFORMATION

Review history

This needs to be brief and to the point in the presence of severe symptoms:

1 **Nature of pain, timing, radiation etc.**
- Pain from EP and ovarian accidents is usually, but not always, unilateral. PID pain is almost always bilateral.
- Shoulder tip pain and rectal discomfort are very suggestive of EP.

2 **Relationship to bowel and bladder habit, menses.**

3 **Date of LMP**
- Determine whether this was normal in timing, duration and heaviness, as light bleeding due to EP may be mistaken for a period.
- "Mittelschmerz" (ovulatory pain) occurs midcycle.

4 **Past surgical, medical or gynaecological problems**
- Previous PID, pelvic surgery and endometriosis are risk factors for EP.

Perform abdominal examination

Peri-hepatitis associated with chlamydial PID may cause right upper quadrant (RUQ) tenderness and guarding ('Fitz-Hugh-Curtis' syndrome).

Pelvic examination

Check for enlarged uterus, adnexal masses, adnexal tenderness and cervical excitation (severe pain on gentle pressure on the cervix). Nodules of endometriosis may be palpable on the uterosacral ligaments.

Cervical excitation is not pathognomic of EP, but it does imply peritoneal irritation in the pouch of Douglas due to blood or pus. The absence of cervical excitation and bilateral adnexal tenderness excludes a diagnosis of acute PID. A Cusco's speculum should be passed to assess the cervix for inflammation and discharge. If indicated, swabs should be taken from the vaginal fornices for general culture and from the endocervix and the urethra for *Chlamydia* and *Gonococcus*.

Consider gynaecological causes of acute abdominal pain

Common causes

Ectopic pregnancy
- ALWAYS CONSIDER EP IN ANY WOMAN OF REPRODUCTIVE AGE WITH ACUTE ABDOMINAL PAIN.
- Pain is usually unilateral, with associated shoulder tip pain, rectal discomfort and dizziness or fainting. Pain often precedes vaginal bleeding which is usually mild.
- Look for tachycardia, hypotension, or a postural blood pressure drop.
- The uterus is usually slightly enlarged, with adnexal tenderness and cervical excitation. An adnexal mass is very rarely present.
- The haemoglobin may be low; pregnancy test will be positive.
- Ultrasound may be normal, show endometrial thickening, free fluid in the pouch of Douglas, an adnexal mass or occasionally a gestational sac with fetal heart activity.
- Detailed management is discussed elsewhere.

Miscarriage
- Pain associated with miscarriage is inevitably associated with vaginal bleeding. It usually occurs after the onset of bleeding and heralds imminent expulsion of the pregnancy products. The pain is felt centrally in the lower abdomen and is colicky in nature.
- Ultrasound assessment is required to confirm viability. If non-viable, scanning will confirm if the process is complete or warrants intervention.
- Detailed management is discussed elsewhere.

Ovarian cyst accident
- Pain is usually unilateral and of sudden onset. It may be intermittent as a cyst torts and de-torts, or constant if due to haemorrhage into the cyst. The pain may be referred to the anterior aspect of the thigh or the buttock.
- Abdominal signs vary depending on the size of the cyst. The uterus will usually be of normal size, and a tender mass is palpable in one of the adnexal regions. Pain and tenderness may prevent adequate examination. Cervical excitation is common in the presence of a cyst accident.
- A mildly raised white count is common (10–$15 \times 10^9/l$).
- Diagnosis is confirmed on ultrasound (remember that a normal-sized ovary may occasionally tort, particularly in pubertal girls and in the post-partum period).
- Management is discussed elsewhere.

Pelvic inflammatory disease
- This is much commoner in women under 25 years of age, unless there has been recent instrumentation of the uterus such as the insertion of an IUCD, surgical termination or occasionally hysteroscopy.
- The pain is (almost) always bilateral in the early stages but may localize to one side, particularly if a tubo-ovarian abscess develops. A purulent vaginal discharge is common, but not universal.
- There may be generalized lower abdominal tenderness with guarding and rebound. The cervix may be inflamed and the uterus is very tender with bilateral adnexal tenderness. Cervical excitation is commonly found.
- The white cell count may be raised but this is not a consistent finding.
- The ESR is very non-specific; a raised CRP may be more discerning for the presence of infection.

Acute Abdominal Pain

- Swabs may grow *Chlamydia, Gonococcus,* anaerobes. Multiple organisms may be involved. Laparoscopy is the current gold standard for diagnosis – many women are initially treated on clinical suspicion.
- Detailed management is discussed elsewhere.

Less common causes

Fibroid related pain

- Fibroids are generally painless. Acute presentation outside of pregnancy is unusual and may imply torsion of a pedunculated fibroid. Differentiation from a torted ovarian cyst may be difficult although ultrasound may help. If pain is acute and severe, laparoscopy may be required.
- At laparotomy, deal with the torted fibroid by ligation and division of the pedicle. Only consider hysterectomy if multiple other fibroids and in women whose family is complete, and who have had adequate time to give informed consent. Acute pain after the menopause should arouse suspicion of infarction associated with malignant change (leiomyosarcoma).
- Fibroid degeneration is unusual outside pregnancy. The pain is usually of sudden onset and is excruciating. There may be associated vomiting. A raised white count is common due to necrosis of the fibroid.
- Ultrasound confirms the presence of fibroids and pressure over the fibroid may worsen the pain, confirming the diagnosis of degeneration.

ACTION PLAN

1 **Admit and manage conservatively**

2 **iv fluids if vomiting**

3 **Opiate analgesia (PCA may be useful)**

4 **Reassure that there is no risk to the pregnancy (although neonatal opiate withdrawal may be a problem if degeneration occurs in late pregnancy)**

5 **Avoid surgery**

Rare causes

Haematocolpos

- Primary amenorrhea associated with lower abdominal pain and a tender central lower abdominal mass. Confirm with external examination of vulva and introitus. Usually in girls under 15 years.

Torsion of other adnexal structures (fimbrial cyst, hydrosalpinx)

- These rare events are likely to be diagnosed at laparoscopy for suspected ovarian cyst torsion. If possible, the ovary should be conserved in premenopausal women if it is not involved. Remember that the Fallopian tube can tort. This is rare and occurs either when there is a hydrosalpinx or when there is an isolated section of tube (e.g. after sterilization or partial salpingectomy).

Ovarian hyperstimulation syndrome
Endometrioma

- May present with cyclical lower abdominal pain. Usually with a deposit within a previous abdominal scar (commonly after Caesarean section).

Haematometra

Occurs in two distinct populations.

- Following endometrial resection, particularly if surgery involved the cervico-isthmic junction. Pain may be cyclical in nature initially. Treatment involves cervical dilatation with hysteroscopy. Repeat resection may become necessary.
- A rarer presentation of post-menopausal bleeding (associated with pain). Confirmed at transvaginal scan or hysteroscopy.

Pyometra

- Presents in the same groups as described for haematometra. Do not always present with pain, but associated purulent vaginal discharge is common.

Consider non-gynaecological causes of acute abdominal pain

This is not an exhaustive list, but should act as a reminder of the many non-gynaecological causes of acute abdominal pain that may present to the gynaecologist.

Remember – NOT EVERYONE PRESENTING AS A GYNAECOLOGICAL EMERGENCY WILL HAVE A GYNAECOLOGICAL CAUSE FOR THEIR PAIN

Surgical causes	Medical causes
Acute appendicitis	Constipation
Ureteric colic/calculi	Urinary tract infection
Diverticular disease	Diverticulitis
Meckel's diverticulum	Inflammatory bowel disease
Cholecystitis	Threadworm infestation
Peptic ulcer disease	Interstitial cystitis
Pancreatitis	Sickle cell crisis
Intestinal obstruction/volvulus	Porphyria
Ruptured liver/spleen	
Subrectus haematoma	
Interstitial cystitis	
Gastrointestinal carcinoma	

REMEMBER TO INVOLVE RELEVANT SURGEON IN THE MANAGEMENT

Investigations (as dictated by clinical situation)

- All women of reproductive age with acute abdominal pain should have a pregnancy test, a FBC and urinalysis. Further investigations will depend on the clinical findings and the results of the above tests.
- Modern urine pregnancy tests will detect hCG at levels of 50 IU/ml (i.e. 2–3 days post-implantation and before a period is missed).
- A negative urine pregnancy test, if properly performed, excludes a symptomatic EP.
- A raised white cell count suggests an inflammatory process such as PID or acute appendicitis, as does an increased C-RP or ESR.

SURGICAL MANAGEMENT OF OVARIAN CYSTS IN THE PREGNANT AND NON-PREGNANT

Olanrewaju Sorinola and Kim Hinshaw

Ovarian cysts are common. They are the fourth most common gynaecological cause of hospital admission and by the age of 65 years, 4% of all women in the UK will have been admitted to hospital for this reason. Ninety percent of all ovarian tumours are benign, although this varies with age. Among surgically managed cases the frequency of malignant tumours is 13% in premenopausal women and 45% in post-menopausal women. Most benign ovarian tumours are cystic, and the finding of solid elements makes malignancy more likely. However, fibromas, thecomas, dermoids and Brenner tumours usually have solid elements. The most common benign tumours associated with pregnancy are mature cystic teratomas (dermoid cysts), which constitute close to 50% in most series. These are bilateral in 12% of cases. The second most common tumours are cystadenomas.

ACTION PLAN

1 **Consider indications for surgical management**
 • Remember – 'THIN RIM`
 • **T** - Torsion
 • **H** - Haemorrhage
 • **I** - Infection
 • **N** – Necrosis
 • **R** - Rupture
 • **I** - Infarction
 • **M** - Malignant change

2 **Consider possible differential diagnoses**

3 **Do a careful and thorough bimanual examination**

4 **Arrange laboratory investigations**

5 **Arrange imaging studies**

6 **Decide on the surgical approach – laparoscopy or laparotomy**

7 **Consider cystectomy, oophorectomy or salpingo-oophorectomy**

8 **Avoid aspiration and fenestration of cysts**

9 **Note special considerations in the pregnant woman**
 • Progesterone or hCG replacement in early pregnancy.
 • Steroids and tocolytics in preterm pregnancy (24–34 weeks).

CONSULT OTHER TOPICS

Acute abdominal pain (p 1)
Other causes of abdominal pain in early pregnancy (p 83)
Scan findings relevant to the Early Pregnancy Assessment Unit (p 68)

SUPPLEMENTARY INFORMATION

Consider indications for surgical management

Emergency surgical management of an ovarian cyst is usually required because of a cyst accident. The patient presents with symptoms due to one of the following: torsion, haemorrhage, rupture or infection. All could present with acute or subacute abdominal pain, tenderness, guarding, rigidity and presence of an adnexal mass accompanied by hypovolaemia or hypotension, leucocytosis and fever. Rapid increase in size should heighten suspicion of haemorrhage into the cyst or malignant change.

Consider possible differential diagnoses

The differential diagnosis of accidents to ovarian cyst (as listed below) is broad, reflecting the wide range of presenting symptoms.

- EP   Appendicitis / Appendix abscess
- Fibroid uterus   Ureteric colic
- Diverticulitis   Pancreatitis
- PID   Hydro- or pyosalpinx

It is sometimes impossible to distinguish between a ruptured bleeding corpus luteum and an EP. Pain originating from the urinary tract, GI tract or its appendages is often confused with pain of gynaecologic origin.

Arrange laboratory investigations

Blood should be sent for FBC, grouping or X-matching. Serum amylase, urea, electrolytes and liver function tests should also be requested. A urine pregnancy test should be done and urine sample sent for microscopy and culture. In premenopausal women, serum CA125 is too non-specific and can be elevated by many other conditions including endometriosis. However, a significantly raised serum CA125 is strongly suggestive of ovarian carcinoma, especially in postmenopausal women.

Arrange imaging studies

Ultrasound is useful in confirming the diagnosis of an ovarian cyst. Apart from revealing the presence of an adnexal mass, it is usually impossible to differentiate between benign and malignant cysts. Features which would suggest malignancy include multilocular appearance, opaque fluid, solid components and papillary projections within the cyst wall, excrescences and the presence of ascites. In ovarian cyst torsion, fluid levels are sometimes seen. However, they can be completely anechoic in other cases, following resorption of the blood. Dermoid cysts have a variable ultrasound appearance ranging from predominantly cystic to a predominantly solid-appearing mass. A haemorrhagic ovarian cyst may easily be misdiagnosed as a pathological mass because of the variable appearance of ultrasonographic images at presentation. A plain film of the abdomen might reveal calcification in cases of dermoid cyst. It may also show air pockets as a result of abscess formation in an infected cyst. The use of computed tomography (CT) scan and magnetic resonance imaging (MRI) as diagnostic aids in cases where ultrasound has failed to provide a definitive diagnosis is quite limited, bearing in mind the acuteness of most presentations.

Decide on the surgical approach – laparoscopy or laparotomy

The standard contraindications to laparoscopy still apply even though the trend these days seems to suggest that a considerable proportion of cases can be managed laparoscopically without compromising the patient's well being. The advantages of laparoscopic surgery are less post-operative pain, shorter hospital stay, quicker return to normal activities and possibly less adhesion formation than after an open procedure.

However, the consequences of spillage of cyst contents, incomplete excision of the cyst wall and an unexpected histological diagnosis of malignancy are considerable disadvantages. Up to 83% of malignant ovarian tumours found by chance at a laparoscopic operation for a 'cyst' are treated inadequately. These operations require considerable expertise in laparoscopic manipulation and should not be attempted without appropriate training, especially in acute emergencies. Nevertheless, even complete torsion of an ovarian cyst has been successfully managed laparoscopically. Successful detorsion and ovarian conservation has been reported.

Consider cystectomy, oophorectomy or salpingo-oophorectomy

In cystectomy, the ovarian capsule is incised and the cyst wall separated from the ovary. The cyst is then removed without dissemination of the contents. In a woman of less than 35 years of age an ovarian cyst is very unlikely to be malignant. Even if the mass is a primary ovarian malignancy, it is likely to be a germ cell tumour, which is responsive to chemotherapy. Thus, ovarian cystectomy or unilateral oophorectomy are safe treatments for unilateral ovarian cysts in this age group with preservation of fertility. Bilateral dysgerminomas are not common, even allowing for microscopic disease in an apparently normal ovary.

Avoid aspiration and fenestration of cysts

Aspiration and fenestration (removal of a window of the cyst wall, for histological analysis) has several disadvantages. Recurrence, spillage of cyst contents and failure to diagnose a malignancy are all possible, even if the inner surface of the cyst is carefully inspected, the fluid sent for cytological assessment and careful peritoneal lavage performed.

Note special considerations in the pregnant woman

Most ovarian cysts in pregnancy are asymptomatic, and are detected on routine ultrasound scan. In early pregnancy, simple unilocular cysts up to 5 cm in diameter are usually luteal cysts. There is no evidence of increased incidence of complications, therefore asymptomatic cases can be dealt with post-natally. If surgery is planned for large cysts during pregnancy, it is best performed at the start of the mid-trimester to reduce the risk of miscarriage. However, if accidents do occur, an urgent operation should not be postponed solely because of pregnancy and dangers of surgery to the fetus. Laparotomy and oophorectomy will usually be required. If the corpus luteum is removed in very early pregnancy, progesterone or human chorionic gonadotrophin can be used as replacement therapy. In later pregnancy, even though the likelihood of labour ensuing is small, steroids should be given as necessary and the operation covered by tocolytic drugs.

FURTHER READING

Russell P and Fansworth A (1997) *Surgical Pathologies of the Ovaries*, 2nd edn. Churchill Livingstone, pp. 155–157.

OVARIAN HYPERSTIMULATION SYNDROME

Niamh McCabe and Kim Hinshaw

Ovarian hyperstimulation syndrome (OHSS) is an iatrogenic condition caused by ovulation induction (OI) for the treatment of infertility, particularly if using hMG with hCG luteal support. Patients with polycystic ovarian disease (PCOD) are at increased risk of developing OHSS. It may be mild (2–6% of OI cycles), moderate or severe (0.1–0.2%) of cycles. The pathogenesis is poorly understood, but the condition is characterized by ovarian enlargement and the shift of fluid from the intravascular space into the peritoneal, pleural and rarely, pericardial spaces. There is resultant oliguria. The increase in capillary permeability may be due to increased production of prostaglandin and histamine. OHSS presents with vague symptoms of headache, nausea, vomiting, dizziness and abdominal pain. All professionals should be aware of the importance of these symptoms in patients undergoing OI. OHSS can be a life-threatening condition and serious thromboembolic complications are not uncommon.

ACTION PLAN

1 **Assess disease severity – clinical, ultrasound and laboratory**
- Mild, moderate or severe disease.
- Baseline weight and abdominal circumference – daily.
- Repeat laboratory assessment daily if admitted.

2 **Arrange admission as appropriate**
- Mild – outpatient care.
- Moderate – admit.
- Severe – admit for HDU/ITU care.

3 **Fluid replacement**

4 **Drainage of collections if symptomatic**

5 **Thromboprophylaxis**
- Enoxaparin 40 mg sc or tinzaparin 3500 IU sc daily.

6 **Analgesia**

7 **Consider co-existing pathology**
- Cyst accident.
- Ectopic.

8 **Consider termination of pregnancy**

9 **Remember complications:**
- Vascular.
- Liver dysfunction.
- Respiratory distress.
- Renal dysfunction.
- Adnexal torsion.

CONSULT OTHER TOPICS

Acute abdominal pain (p 1)
Surgical management of ovarian cysts in the pregnant and non-pregnant (p 6)

SUPPLEMENTARY INFORMATION

Assess disease severity

Several different classifications have been suggested. The Golan classification is clinically based. It involves objective ultrasound criteria as well as clinical condition and laboratory changes.

Mild

- Grade 1 – abdominal distension and discomfort.
- Grade 2 – features of grade 1 plus nausea, vomiting +/– diarrhoea; ovaries enlarged 5–12 cm.

Moderate

- Grade 3 – features of mild OHSS plus scan evidence of ascites.

Severe

- Grade 4 – features of moderate OHSS plus clinical evidence of ascites +/– hydrothorax and breathing difficulties.
- Grade 5 – all of the above plus alteration in blood volume, increased viscosity (related to haemoconcentration), coagulation defects and reduced renal perfusion and function.

Take blood for FBC, haematocrit (Hct), coagulation studies, urea and electrolytes, liver function tests – repeat daily. Perform pregnancy test (disease is worse in conception cycles). Perform abdominal ultrasound for ovarian size. Arrange chest X-ray. Consider echocardiography.

Mild disease with minimal symptoms, normal Hct and minimally enlarged ovaries (<5 cm) may be managed on an outpatient basis with simple analgesia and increased oral fluids. Allow direct access to ward if condition deteriorates.

Moderate and severe disease require hospital admission. Severe disease (Hct >45%, WCC >15 000/ml, oliguria, ovarian size >12 cm) requires HDU or ITU admission.

Involve specialists in other disciplines – anaesthetics, cardiology and nephrology will be required in severe cases.

Fluid replacement

Strict fluid balance is essential and a central venous pressure line is necessary in severe disease to assess response to iv therapy. Urinary catheterization is required.

Crystalloid solution should be used initially, but consider colloid in the presence of Hct >45%, worsening ascites or hypoalbuminaemia (<30 g/dl). Avoid diuretics as circulating volume is already reduced.

Drainage of collections if symptomatic

Tense ascites may lead to respiratory embarrassment, may affect renal function by compression of the renal veins or may reduce venous return by compression of the IVC. Drainage may be necessary in these situations or to relieve symptoms.

Paracentesis must be under ultrasound guidance to avoid damage to the enlarged ovaries, and may be done TV. Pleurocentesis may be necessary to improve respiratory function. Cardiac tamponade is a recognized complication and requires drainage. Drainage procedures may need repeating.

Analgesia

NSAIDs are contraindicated as they may precipitate renal failure by their action on renal prostaglandins (vasodilator PGs maintain renal circulation in the face of hypovolaemia). Simple analgesics such as paracetamol may be used, with or without codeine. If these are ineffective, parenteral opiates will be required.

If pain is severe, consider co-existing pathology (see next paragraph).

Consider co-existing pathology

Severe pain may indicate a cyst accident such as haemorrhage or torsion, or even EP. Diagnosis may be difficult in the presence of ascites and enlarged ovaries.

Any surgical procedure must be carried out by senior personnel because the ovaries in OHSS are extremely friable and respond poorly to handling. Consider laparoscopic de-torting of ovarian cyst. Avoid laparotomy if possible.

Consider termination

OHSS usually improves in the luteal phase of the index cycle and resolves by day 20–40. In conception cycles, it may persist and complications are more likely. Interruption of the pregnancy may be necessary to safeguard the health of the mother.

Remember complications

- Vascular
  1. Cerebrovascular accident.
  2. Peripheral embolization – loss of limbs reported.
  3. Thrombophlebitis/DVT.
- Liver dysfunction
- Respiratory distress (pleural effusion)
- Cardiovascular compromise (pericardial effusion)
- Renal dysfunction
- Adnexal torsion

FURTHER READING

Brinsden P, Wada I, Tan SL, Balen A, Jacobs HS (1995) Diagnosis, prevention and management of ovarian hyperstimulation syndrome. *BJOG* **102:** 767–772.

Rizk B (1994) Ovarian hyperstimulation syndrome. In: Studd J (Ed.) *Progress in Obstetrics and Gynaecology*, Volume 11. Churchill Livingstone, London, pp. 311–341.

UPPER TRACT PELVIC INFECTION

Keith Allenby and Kim Hinshaw

Upper genital tract infection or pelvic inflammatory disease (PID) is a common gynaecological emergency. The disease ranges from relatively asymptomatic endocervical infection, through endometritis, endosalpingitis, to pelvic peritonitis and tubo-ovarian abscess. Action plans are presented for the management of pelvic infection presenting on an emergency basis:

1. Diagnostic laparosocopy in acute PID.
2. Tubo-ovarian abscess.
3. Endometritis and secondary postpartum haemorrhage.

The management of infection complicating miscarriage and therapeutic abortion is discussed in detail in other sections in this book. Diagnosis and appropriate treatment is extremely important if we are to avoid the long-term sequelae of pelvic infection, namely chronic pelvic pain, EP and tubal subfertility. With the emergence of HIV, unusual types of pelvic infection such as tuberculosis, are becoming more common. The association of PID with other genital tract infection must be considered and appropriate follow up with genito-urinary medicine colleagues should be arranged where appropriate.

DIAGNOSTIC LAPAROSCOPY IN ACUTE PELVIC INFECTION

1 **Review history**

2 **Examination**
- Abdominal and pelvic.

3 **Investigation**
- Endocervical swabs (C&S, gonococcus, chlamydia).
- High vaginal swab (HVS).
- FBC (WCC).
- ESR or C-RP.
- Urinary hCG.
- Consider LFTs (if RUQ pain).
- Consider pelvic ultrasound.

4 **Indications for laparoscopy**
- Significant PID not settling with iv antibiotics (may proceed to laparotomy).
- Need to exclude other pathology (ectopic, cyst accident, appendicitis etc.).
- Laparoscopy is still the diagnostic 'gold standard' and allows direct specimen collection for culture.

5 **Laparoscopy in acute pelvic infection**
- Double-puncture technique required to adequately visualize all pelvic organs.
- Check tubal, ovarian and uterine mobility, damage, adhesions etc.
- Obtain free fuid, exudate etc. for culture.
- Visualize liver – exclude perihepatitis ('Fitz-Hugh-Curtis`).

6 **Subsequent treatment**
- If clinically indicated – appropriate antibiotic cover *before* culture results.
- Remove IUCD in mild disease if symptoms not settled in 24–48 hours.

7 **Follow up**
- Outpatient review if significant pelvic damage suspected (tubal damage = 8% – 1 episode, 19.5% – 2 episodes, 40% – 3 episodes).
- Consider referral of patient and partner for GUM assessment.

CONSULT OTHER TOPICS

Acute abdominal pain (p 1)
Complications of the intrauterine contraceptive device (p 42)
Ectopic pregnancy (p 76)

SUPPLEMENTARY INFORMATION

Review history

The incidence of chlamydia is rising in the younger sexually active age group. Common presenting symptoms are irregular menstrual bleeding with associated vague lower abdominal pain and vaginal discharge. Recent gynaecological surgery (hysteroscopy, IUCD insertion, laparoscopy, termination, ERPC etc.) may be a positive risk factor. Menstruation increases the risk of ascending infection. As disease severity increases, pain worsens, with systemic upset and developing signs of pelvic peritonitis. EP should always be considered.

Examination and investigation

Assess general condition. Look for signs of abdominal and pelvic peritonism/peritonitis ('cervical excitation'). Exclude obvious pelvic mass ('tubo-ovarian'). Right upper quadrant pain may indicate 'Fitz-Hugh-Curtis' syndrome (perihepatitis, particularly associated with chlamydial infection – perihepatic adhesions; occasionally abnormal LFTs).
    Remove IUCD in moderate or severe infection.

Subsequent treatment

If systemically unwell, antibiotic cover is required for chlamydia, anaerobes and *Neisseria gonorrhoea*:

- iv gentamicin, metronidazole and penicillin.

Oral preparations:
- Metronidazole 400 mg 8 hourly for 7 days with one of the three following drugs:
    1. Erythromycin 500 mg 6 hourly for 14 days or
    2. Doxycycline 100 mg 12 hourly for 14 days or
    3. Azithromycin 1.2 g stat single dose.

TUBO-OVARIAN ABSCESS

ACTION PLAN

1 Review history
- Patient is likely to be systemically ill.
- Care if observations deteriorate despite aggressive iv antibiotics.

2 Examination and investigation
- May suggest tender abdomino-pelvic mass.
- Blood cultures may be indicated.

3 Indications for laparoscopy/laparotomy
- Clinical condition deteriorating.
- Inadequate response to conservative management with iv antibiotics.
- Diagnosis remains unclear after appropriate investigation.

4 Laparotomy for tubo-ovarian abscess
- iv antibiotic cover.
- Prophylactic heparin cover.
- Incision which allows adequate access.
- Consider vertical incision if diagnosis unclear or large/complex mass.
- Define abscess – open and drain pus.
- Break down all locules digitally.
- Divide adhesions which limit access to the mass or which tether bowel.
- Careful lavage of peritoneal cavity at the end of the procedure.
- DO NOT TRY TO EXCISE THE MASS – may lead to difficulty maintaining haemostasis.
- Leave large bore drain into abscess cavity/pelvis.

5 Subsequent treatment
- Continue iv antibiotics until situation is resolving (24–48 hours).
- Appropriate analgesia.
- Watch for paralytic ileus.

6 Follow up
- Consider outpatient review (particularly if fertility is an issue).

CONSULT OTHER TOPIC

Septic shock (p 267)

OTHER INFECTIONS

Tuberculosis

TB is not a true ascending pelvic infection, but is always secondary to another source woth haematogenous spread. Incidence is rising related to the incidence of HIV. Consider the diagnosis in patients with weight loss, anorexia and night sweats in association with the following gynaecological symptoms: subfertility (classic 'pipe stem' at HSG with calcification), pelvic mass, chronic pelvic pain, menorrhagia, amenorrhoea, vaginal discharge. Patients may be asymptomatic.

Diagnosis confirmed by long-term culture or Ziehl-Neelsen stain (use late secretory endometrium). In view of developing drug resistance, treatment will be co-ordinated by physicians with an interest in infectious disease.

Actinomycosis

Actinomycosis israelii is a gram positive mycelium-bearing anaerobic fungus, associated with the presence of the IUCD. Incidence increases relative to the time the coil has been *in situ* (particularly inert coils). Commonly detected in cervical smears in asymptomatic women, but can rarely present with major pelvic abscess.

If asymptomatic – consider coil change to copper-based system. If symptomatic (pain, discharge, dyspareunia) – remove coil and give prolonged course of high-dose oral penicillin.

ENDOMETRITIS AND SECONDARY POST-PARTUM HAEMORRHAGE

ACTION PLAN

1 Review history
- Classically admitted within 14 days of delivery.
- Increasing lochia +/– abdominal pain.
- Review maternity notes ref: delivery etc.

2 Examination and investigation
- Confirm appropriate involution of uterus – examine cervical os (?open).
- If haemodynamically *unstable* (unusual) – institute ABCs of resuscitation.
- FBC (WCC).
- Group and hold (X-match adequately if indicated).
- Blood cultures (if T 38.5°C).
- Endocervical swabs.
- Consider urinary hCG (to exclude rare possibility of GTD).

3 Initial management
- If stable (majority) – manage as likely 'endometritis':
  1. Broad spectrum antibiotic cover (oral or iv as clinically indicated).
  2. Maintain hydration.
  3. Conservative approach – majority will settle within 24 hours.
  4. Discharge with 7 day course of antibiotics to complete.
- If very heavy bleeding on admission:
  1. Investigations as above.
  2. Consider ergometrine.
  3. Consider intrauterine ballon tamponade (500 ml 'Rusch' urological balloon).
  4. May need to consider *careful* haemostatic curettage.
  5. Senior staff should be in theatre for the procedure.

4 Subsequent treatment
- Conservative management (with antibiotics) will settle the majority.
- Ultrasound assessment is not routinely required – reserve for those cases who do not respond to initial conservative management. Remember that ultrasound does not differentiate well between blood clot, decidua and placental tissue. The results must be interpreted with care in planning potential surgical intervention.

FURTHER READING

RCOG Pace Review 98/04 (1998) *Pelvic inflammatory disease*. RCOG, London.

VULVAL AND LOWER TRACT GENITAL INFECTION

David Evans and Kim Hinshaw

Lower genital tract infections are very common and patients present to both gynae-cologists and genito-urinary medicine (GUM) specialists. Most GUM services offer open access and allow self-referral. Severe lower genital tract infection will often present to the Accident and Emergency Department or as a gynaecological emergency. In this chapter we present action plans for the management of the following infections which may present on an emergency basis:

- Acute infection of Bartholin's gland.
- Vulval/labial abscess.
- Acute herpes vulvitis.
- Acute vulvo-vaginal candidiasis.

The gynaecologist should also be aware of the many forms of lower genital tract infection which present on a semi-urgent basis, often with symptoms of discharge, bleeding and/or occasionally localized pain. Remember that these infections may also infect the lower urinary tract (in particular, the urethra) and the perianal/rectal area:

- Bacterial vaginosis.
- Ano-genital warts.
- Vaginal warts.
- Chlamydia.
- Trichomonas.
- Syphilis.
- Gonorrhoea.

ACUTE INFECTION OF BARTHOLIN'S GLAND

ACTION PLAN

1 **Take history**
- Short history of swelling of the base of the labia majora.
- Increasing pain.
- May give a prior history of painful episodes attentuated by antibiotics.
- Consider systemic disease if recurrent abscess (e.g. diabetes).

2 **Examination**

3 **Avoid antibiotics**
- Do not give antibiotics if there is an obvious mass.
- This may lead to partial treatment but rarely resolution.

4 **Arrange surgical drainage**
- Verbal discussion of procedure and obtain written consent.

5 **Drainage of abscess and marsupialization**
- General anaesthetic is usually recommended.
- Lithotomy position with adequate exposure and good lighting.
- Take swabs *before* aseptic preparation.
- Make a deep cruciate incison over the abscess (2–3 cm in horizontal and

vertical directions). Ideally at lower aspect of vulva, outside hymenal ring at point of drainage of duct.

- Allow pus to drain.
- Break down all internal locules digitally.
- Excise the skin flaps with scissors – create a round hole 2–3 cm in diameter.
- Identify the internal abscess/gland wall within the line of the incision.
- Use interrupted absorbable polyglycolic acid/polyglactin sutures to attach the edge of the gland wall to the skin surface (x 6–8 will usually be required). This creates a 'pouch` (i.e. gland is marsupialized).
- Pack the cavity with a moistened ribbon gauze.

6 **Post-operative management and advice**

- Remove pack at 12–24 hours.
- Further antibiotics are not routinely required (check swabs for gonorrhoea).
- Offer advice on local hygiene.
- Advise to keep marsupialized entrance open to allow healing from within (i.e. introduce tip of little finger daily for first few days).

SUPPLEMENTARY INFORMATION

Examination

Systemic effects are unusual (e.g. fever). Adequate examination is usually not possible because of significant tenderness. A tense, unilateral, inflamed swelling is seen at the base of the affected labium majorum (usually appears 4–5 cm in diameter). This is misleading as the abscess cavity may extend anteriorly into the labium and 8–10 cm posteriorly into the ischio-rectal fat. Examination is not usually required until general anaesthetic has been administered. Opiates may be required if surgery is deferred for any reason (e.g. until daylight hours).

Arrange surgical drainage

The Bartholin's gland is a poor anatomical design. It is a large structure draining a thick secretion through a small duct. It lies in an area exposed to friction/trauma with a surrounding rich, commensal bacterial flora. Surgical drainage aims to:

- relieve pain;
- release pus;
- breakdown abscess loculations;
- prevent recurrence by allowing free drainage to the skin surface.

Swabs should be taken before aseptic preparation, as up to 25% of cases have been reported to be +ve for *Gonococcus*.

VULVAL/LABIAL ABSCESS

ACTION PLAN

1 **Take history**
- May give a history of previous painful episodes settling on antibiotics (particularly if related to infected sebaceous gland/hair follicles).
- Consider systemic disease if recurrent abscess (e.g. diabetes).

2 **Examination**
- Discrete, fluctuant mass in labia or hair-bearing areas of vulva/mons pubis.
- More anteriorly placed than Bartholin's abscess.

3 **Antibiotics**
- A trial of broad-spectrum antibiotics (including flucloxacillin or erythromycin) may be beneficial if the lesion is <2 cm and area is indurated *without* a discrete mass.

4 **Arrange surgical drainage**
- Verbal discussion of procedure and obtain written consent.

5 **Drainage of abscess**
- General anaesthetic is usually recommended.
- Lithotomy position with adequate exposure and good lighting.
- Make a deep cruciate incision over the abscess (2–3 cm in horizontal and vertical directions dependent on size of abscess).
- Allow pus to drain.
- Break down any internal locules digitally.
- Consider packing the cavity with a moistened ribbon gauze.
- Suturing of individual bleeding vessels in incision edges is rarely required.

6 **Post-operative management and advice**
- Remove pack at 12–24 hours.
- Antibiotics are not routinely required unless systemically ill or if significant spreading erythema/cellulitis.
- Offer advice on local hygiene.

ACUTE PRIMARY HERPES VULVITIS

ACTION PLAN

1 **Take history**
- Blistering and ulceration – vulva, cervix, rectum.
- Severe vulval pain/dysuria.
- Local lymphadenopathy.
- Vaginal/urethral discharge.
- Systemic symptoms.

2 **Examination**
- Take swabs from base of lesions (remember – acutely tender!).

3 **Antivirals**
- Start within 5 days of symptoms or whilst new lesions appearing. Treatment for 5 days to reduce severity and duration of attack:
  1. Aciclovir 200 mg x 5 daily.

2. Famciclovir 250 mg x 3 daily.

3. Valaciclovir 500 mg x 2 daily.

- iv dosing available if systemically ill and cannot take oral.

4 Analgesia

- Avoid topical local anaesthetic – high risk of sensitization.
- Otherwise give adequate analgesia (dihydrocodeine, diclofenac, opiates).

5 Antibiotics

- May be required if secondary bacterial infection (consider flucloxacillin).

6 Catheterization

- Suprapubic route is preferable.

7 GUM referral and follow-up

- Initial opinion may be sought during acute admission.
- GUM follow-up recommended for patient and partner.
- Advise about secondary attacks.
- Advise about pregnancy-related issues.

CONSULT OTHER TOPIC

Acute retention of urine (p 141)

SUPPLEMENTARY INFORMATION

History

Usual agent is herpes simplex virus type II but can be caused by type I ('cold sore' virus). The primary attack is the most painful. Systemic effects include fever, myalgia, autonomic neuropathy and meningitis. Severe pain may lead to presentation with acute urinary retention.

Examination

Only superficial examination is possible because of significant tenderness. Classical lesions may be seen on the vulva. There is often associated oedema, inflammation and there may also be secondary bacterial infection. Virus is labile, so appropriate swabs should be transported directly to laboratory (culture has >90% sensitivity and high specificity).

ACUTE VULVO-VAGINAL CANDIDIASIS

ACTION PLAN

1 **Take history**
- Vaginal discharge.
- Pruritis vulvae.
- Superficial dyspareunia.
- Vulval pain.

2 **Examination**
- Vulval erythema/fissuring oedema.
- Satellite lesions – inner thighs and abdomen.
- Vaginal discharge – like 'cottage cheese'.

3 **Diagnosis**
- Microscopy – gram stain for spores and pseudohyphae.
- Swabs.

4 **Treatment**
- Topical or oral Azole therapies (80–95% cure rates).

5 **Analgesia**
- Adequate analgesia may be required in severe vulvovaginitis (dihydrocodeine, diclofenac, rarely opiates).

6 **GUM referral and follow-up**
- Initial opinion may be sought if admitted acutely.
- GUM follow-up recommended if recurrent infections (species typing).
- Anti-mycotics are fungi-static rather than fungicidal. Prolonged therapy may be necessary for recurrent infection:
  1. Fluconazole 100 mg weekly for 6 months.
  2. Clotrimazole pessaries 500 mg weekly for 6 months.
  3. Itraconazole 400 mg monthly for 6 months.
  4. Ketoconazole 100 mg daily for 6 months.

FURTHER READING

Barton SE (2000) Classification, general principles of vulval infections. *Curr. Obstet. Gynaecol.* **10:** 2–6.

Rogers CA and Beardell AJ (1999) Recurrent vulvovaginal candidiasis. *Int. J. STD AIDS* **10:** 435–441.

TOXIC SHOCK SYNDROME

Niamh McCabe and Kim Hinshaw

Toxic shock syndrome (TSS) was originally described in children and teenagers, but is now widely thought of as a gynaecological condition. It is probably due to the effects of an exotoxin produced by *Staphylococcus aureus* ('toxic shock syndrome toxin' or TSST-1). Occasionally Group A, β *Haemolytic streptococci* can cause similar systemic disturbance related to toxin secretion ('erythrogenic toxin A'). There is a strong association with menstruation and the use of tampons, especially those with very high absorbency, but can occur in other situations including post-partum.

TSS presents with a sudden high fever, muscle pains and a widespread rash that looks like sunburn and desquamates after 7–10 days. Mortality remains significant but has fallen from 15% to 3%. A high index of suspicion is required – the condition should be considered in the differential diagnosis of any young woman who presents with rash and/or fever who is systemically ill or unstable.

ACTION PLAN

1 If shocked on admission – resuscitate, establish venous access etc.

2 Consider suspicious symptoms and signs
- Look for the classic rash.
- Fever, myalgia, diarrhoea and vomiting.
- Hypotension.

3 Arrange blood investigations
- FBC, U&Es, LFTs, glucose and creatinine kinase.
- Group and save, clotting screen.
- Blood cultures.

4 Perform vaginal examination
- Take swabs (including HVS) for C&S.
- Remove tampon if present (*thorough* speculum examination is needed).

5 Administer appropriate β-lactamase resistant antibiotic:
- Flucloxacillin 1 g 6 hourly iv.
- Cefuroxime 1.5 g 6 hourly iv.
- Discuss case with Consultant Microbiologist.

6 Transfer to ITU
- Inotropic support may be required.
- Manage as per septic shock.

CONSULT OTHER TOPICS

Anaphylaxis (p 240)
Cardiopulmonary resuscitation (p 234)
Septic shock (p 267)
Vulval and lower tract genital infection (p 17)

SUPPLEMENTARY INFORMATION

If shocked on admission – resuscitate, establish venous access etc.

There is often only a short prodromal phase with non-specific symptoms of malaise or diarrhoea. Vaginal discharge may be noted. More often the patient will show symptoms and signs of generalized systemic illness or even septic shock.

Consider suspicious symptoms and signs

The rash is often diffusely distributed with blanching erythema and areas of oedema. When desquamation occurs, it typically affects the palms and soles. Pyrexia is abrupt in onset and significant ($\geq 39°C$) and muscular pains are common. Respiratory compromise implies severe disease.

TSS has been described in association with necrotizing fasciitis, burns, excision of skin lesions and after endometrial resection.

Arrange blood investigations

A high white count and reduced platelets are common with changes in liver function including raised bilirubin. Creatinine phosphokinase may be increased. As disease progresses and multi-organ involvement occurs, renal function may be impaired and DIC may develop. Blood cultures should be taken but may be negative.

Administer appropriate β-lactamase resistant antibiotic

Often, aggressive triple iv antibiotic therapy will be recommended by the microbiologist in order to cover other possible causes of septic shock; β-lactamase resistant drugs should be included if TSS is a possibility. TSS can relapse at menstruation and in the puerperium. In the latter case it has been associated with clostridial organisms. The use of tampons should be avoided until *Staphylococcus aureus* has been eradicated from the vagina.

Transfer to ITU

The presentation may be very similar to septic shock consequent on any other cause of bacteraemia or septicaemia (i.e. hypotension and respiratory compromise and potential multi-organ dysfunction syndrome (MODS)). Intensive supportive management is detailed in the chapter on septic shock. Involvement of an intensive care specialist at an early stage is vital.

FURTHER READING

Todd J, Fishant M, Kapral F and Welch T (1978) Toxic shock syndrome associated with phage group 1 staphylococci. *Lancet* **ii:** 1116–1118.

Toxic Shock Syndrome

GENITAL TRACT TRAUMA

Helen Cameron and Niamh McCabe

Genital tract trauma may vary from minor vaginal abrasions due to consensual sexual activity to life-threatening pelvic damage from impalement. When assessing a woman with trauma to the genital tract, it is important to remember that she may be too embarrassed to give a full history of the causative incident and that 'vaginal bleeding' may signify extensive damage to extravaginal sites. The examining doctor may need to consider the possibility of sexual assault and raise the issue with the patient.

Examination may be accepted in the emergency department or on the gynaecology ward. Consideration must be given to offering examination under anaesthetic, particularly if the trauma is significant and/or bleeding continues. This is often required for children, even with minor genital tract trauma.

CAUSES OF GENITAL TRAUMA

These can be categorized as:

- Genital trauma due to voluntary sexual activity.
- Unintentional genital injury – prepubertal: (a) accidental; (b) due to sexual assault.
- Unintentional genital injury – adult: (a) accidental; (b) due to sexual assault.

Injuries during voluntary sexual activity commonly affect the posterior aspects of the introital area. Tears during first intercourse are usually lower vaginal. Penile injury in the upper vagina does occur, more commonly at the right side of the vault. Minor mucosal injuries can also affect the anorectal area. Vaginal insufflation in pregnancy (orogenital sex) can lead to death from air embolism.

Hymenal disruption in childhood should suggest sexual abuse. Accidental trauma is often perineal ranging from simple 'straddle' injuries to extensive disruption associated with crushing pelvic fracture. In the adult, straddle injuries related to cycling accidents are more likely. Severe trauma may be caused by RTAs, impalement, sport-related trauma (e.g. water-skiing, water-slides etc.), illegal abortion procedures and gunshot/knife wounds. Munchausen's syndrome may present with genital trauma.

ASSOCIATED INJURIES

May involve the bony pelvis, any of the organs within the pelvis (including bladder, urethra, anus/rectum, blood vessels) and intra-abdominal structures (penetrating injuries may damage bowel). Systematic assessment is helped by considering whether injuries are:

- Simple.
- Complex.
- Extensive.

COMPLICATIONS OF GENITAL TRAUMA

May be acute, but injury can also lead to long-term sequelae:

- Haemorrhage: Revealed or hidden (intraperitoneal or retroperitoneal).

- Infection:
  - (a) Local (including pelvic infection, urinary or osteomyelitis).
  - (b) Occasionally systemic.
- Gynaecological:
  - (a) Chronic pelvic pain.
  - (b) Dyspareunia.
  - (c) Infertility.
- Psychological: May need formal counselling (including psychosexual).

CONSULT OTHER TOPICS

Childhood emergencies (p 47)
Female genital mutilation (circumcision or infibulation) (p 28)
Haemorrhage control (p 197)
Management of the rape victim (p 30)

MANAGEMENT OF EXTENSIVE GENITAL TRAUMA

ACTION PLAN

1 **Resuscitate as indicated – follow ABCs**

2 **Brief history and assess likely level of damage**

3 **Catheterize**
- Look for haematuria.
- The inability to pass a catheter suggests urethral injury – consider supra-pubic drainage.

4 **Analgesia**

5 **Examine carefully:**
- Abdomen.
- Vagina (both digitally and with speculum).
- Rectum (include proctoscopy).
- Pelvic girdle.

6 **Check FBC, urinalysis. Consider U&E, group and save. X-match if pelvic fracture**

7 **Abdominal X-ray (erect)**
- Look for free gas – consider perforation of viscus.
- Look for foreign body in vagina or abdomen.

8 **Pelvic X-ray**
- Look for pelvic fracture if RTA or similar.

9 **Pelvic and abdominal ultrasound**
- Look for free fluid, masses, haematoma.

10 **If stable – consider CT/MRI of pelvis if extensive pelvic damage**

11 **Consider EUA +/– cystoscopy +/– sigmoidoscopy**

12 **Involve specialists as required:**
- Anaesthetic.
- Surgical.

- Urological.
- Colorectal.
- Orthopaedic.

13 **Consider iv antibiotics (e.g. cefuroxime 750 mg and metronidazole 500 mg, both iv 8 hourly or amoxycillin/potassium clavulanate 1.2 g iv 6–8 hourly)**

14 **Consider tetanus prophylaxis**

VAGINAL LACERATIONS

ACTION PLAN

1 **Resuscitate and examine as above**

2 **Consider iv antibiotic prophylaxis (see above – single dose may suffice)**

3 **If not actively bleeding, and no evidence of other injury**
- Analgesia.
- Temporary avoidance of sexual intercourse.

4 **If bleeding or extent of injury unclear**
- EUA.

5 **General, epidural or spinal anaesthesia will be required**

6 **Full digital and speculum examination**

7 **Consider proctoscopy if rectum involved. Assess anal sphincters**

8 **Repair of laceration using absorbable glycolide suture in layers**

9 **Consider vaginal pack if extensive minor vaginal lacerations**

10 **Foley catheter while pack *in-situ*. Remove pack in 24 hours**

VULVAL HAEMATOMA

This is the commonest genital trauma seen in practice, usually as the result of an accidental straddle injury (e.g. child slips astride the edge of the bath).

ACTION PLAN

1 **Consider sexual abuse**
- If minor, seek senior paediatric advice and D/W senior gynaecologist.

2 **Gentle examination**

3 **Conservative management can be considered *in adults* if:**
- Not expanding.
- Product of two maximum diameters <15 cm.

There is evidence that vulval/vaginal haematomas larger than this should be surgically drained (reducing recovery time, admission time, need for later surgery)

4 **For large or rapidly expanding haematoma:**
- Examine under anaesthesia.
- Incise vaginal/vulval skin over haematoma.
- Evacuate clot digitally.
- Diathermize or ligate any obvious bleeding vessels (rarely found).
- Corrugated drain if large cavity – exit via skin incision. Secure with suture.
- Leave appropriate opening in incision to allow drainage.
- Consider vaginal pack and catheter if extension para-vaginally.
- iv antibiotics (see above).
- Remove pack after 24 hours.

5 **Even if no catheter used – close observation as urinary retention common**

6 **Reassure patient and family that resolution will be complete with no long-term sequelae**

REFERENCE

Benrubi G, Neuman C, Nuss RC and Thompson RJ (1987) Vulvar and vaginal haematomas: a retrospective study of conservative versus operative management. *South Med. J.* **80(8)**: 991–994.

FEMALE GENITAL MUTILATION (CIRCUMCISION OR INFIBULATION)

Charles Cox

INTRODUCTION

The number of women world-wide who have undergone female circumcision is thought to be between 100 and 140 million with a further 2 million girls at risk.

The groups at risk are from Eritrea, Ethiopia, Somalia and the Yemen. In the UK there are little reliable data. One estimate was that 10 000 girls and young women are at risk and another 3000–4000 new cases occur each year. Many of these young women will be taken abroad for this to carried out. The extent of the procedure varies between excision of the prepuce of the clitoris and full circumcision with removal of the clitoris and labia minora.

IMMEDIATE HEALTH RISKS

These include haemorrhage, severe pain, infections including tetanus, septicaemia and even death.

LATER HEALTH RISKS

Difficulties with micturition. Stenosis of the introitus can lead to virtual obliteration of the introitus with dribbling incontinence and recurrent urinary infections. Fistulae may occur from damage and infection associated with the circumcision procedure. Keloid scars and large inclusion dermoid cysts can occur in the perineum which may cause problems with childbirth.

Problems with menstruation may arise with difficulty of drainage of menstrual fluid leading to pelvic infection.

Problems of fertility are much increased and maternal and perinatal mortality are significantly increased (maternal twice and perinatal four times).

ACTION PLAN

1 **Suspect if a woman from a high-risk areas complains of urinary problems, pelvic pain and problems with menstruation**

2 **Ask the question – 'Have you been circumcised?'**

3 **Examine to confirm the diagnosis and the extent of the procedure**

4 **Discuss reversal**

DISCUSS REVERSAL

In some communities reversal is carried out immediately after marriage. It can be carried out in the later stages of labour but is best done before pregnancy. It should of course be carried out under appropriate anaesthesia.

ACTION PLAN

1 **Place the patient in lithotomy**

2 **Identify the vaginal opening and gently dilate until a probe can be placed under the bridge of skin**

3 **Local infiltration with adrenaline and local anaesthetic may be useful as well as proper anaesthesia**

4 **The tissues are divided in the mid-line and haemostasis achieved. The urethra is identified and exposed**

LEGAL ASPECTS

The Prohibition of Female Circumcision Act (1985) states that it is illegal to repair the labia in such a way as to make intercourse difficult or impossible. This applies particularly to the repair of episiotomies after childbirth when doctors may be asked to restore the circumcision.

REFERENCE

Female Genital Mutilation: caring for patients and child protection. Guidance from the British Medical Association. Approved by Council January 1996 Revised April 2001

USEFUL ADDRESSES

Foundation for Women's Research and Development (FORWARD), 6th Floor, 50, Eastbourne Terrace, London W2 6LX. Tel: 020 7725 2606. Fax: 020 7725 2796. E-mail: forward @dircon.co.uk. Website: www.forward.dircon.co.uk

International Planned Parenthood Federation, Regent's College, Inner Circle, Regent's Park, London NW1 4NS. Tel: 020 7487 7900. Fax: 020 7487 7950. E-mail: info@ippf.org. Website: www.ippf.org

Black Women's Health and Family Support (BWHFS), 82 Russia Lane, London E2 9LU. Tel: 020 8980 3503. Fax: 020 8980 3503. E-mail: lbwhap@dial.pipex.com

MANAGEMENT OF THE RAPE VICTIM

Susan J Houghton

Rape is defined as '*unlawful sexual intercourse by a man with a woman, by force, fear or fraud*' (Sexual Offences Act 1956, England). The man must either know that the woman did not give consent or was reckless (i.e. 'did not care') whether she gave consent or not (Sexual Offences [Amendments] Act 1976, England). This chapter will highlight the role of the examining doctor (forensic medical examiner or FME) in the assessment of victims of sexual assault (the complainant). It will detail the physical and psychological sequelae of rape, what forensic evidence should be obtained, the legal implications of the forensic medical examination and what is required in the witness statement.

THE EXAMINATION OF AN ALLEGED RAPE VICTIM

The victim of sexual assault should be allowed to choose the gender of the examining doctor. The forensic medical examination should take place as soon as possible after the alleged assault and a trained woman police officer should be present. A second examination should be performed 24–48 hours later to find evidence of new bruising or injury and to compare the age of different bruises.

1 **Management of the immediate medical needs of the complainant**
- Injuries requiring immediate medical attention take priority over forensic sampling.
- Treatment should be performed in an appropriate setting (e.g. an accident and emergency department, a specific rape crisis unit or a psychiatric unit).

2 **Accurate history taking of the alleged incident to determine which forensic samples should be taken (see *Table 1*)**
- The FME must be objective and non-judgmental.
- The FME should ask direct questions based upon the first account obtained by the police officer.
- The question and answers should be recorded verbatim in the medical records.

3 **Taking of relevant medical and sexual history (see *Table 2*)**

4 **Obtaining informed consent for:**
- A medical examination – non-genital/genital.
- Collection of forensic evidence.
- Retention of relevant items of clothing for forensic examination.
- Disclosure of details of medical record to the police/Crown Prosecution Service (CPS).

5 **Undertake a systematic forensic medical examination**

6 **Photo-documentation of bites, bruises or other injuries**
- Complex injuries should be photographed.
- Genital or intimate photographs should be taken by a photographer of the same gender.

7 **Collection of forensic samples (see *Table 3*)**
- All swabs are taken in pairs, as well as control swabs (unopened plain swabs from the same batch).
- Bite marks should be swabbed to obtain samples of the assailant's saliva.

8 **Careful labelling and packaging of the samples**
- Transport of specimens to the Forensic Science Laboratory is the responsibility of the police officer present.

9 **Relevant prophylactic therapy**
- Post-coital contraception must be administered if there is a risk of pregnancy – hormonal up to 72 hours (Levonelle 2) or an IUCD up to 5 days after the incident.
- Antibiotics for penetrating bite wounds or infected skin abrasions.

10 **Referral to the GUM Clinic for screening for STDs, HIV, and prophylaxis where indicated**

11 **Follow-up to exclude pregnancy and provide counselling if pregnant**

12 **Referral for appropriate counselling at the time of and after the examination**
- To provide support to the complainant, her spouse, family and friends.
- To treat the sequelae of rape trauma syndrome.
- Rape crisis centres, victim support groups and social workers can provide support.

13 **Completion of a 'professional witness' statement**

14 **Professionals involved should be aware of 'rape trauma syndrome'**

Table 1. Assault history to be taken by FME

Complainant's details
- Name, age, date of birth
- Date, time and place of examination
- Persons present at the examination and their relationship to the victim
- Details of her General Practitioner

Details of the assault
- Date and time of assault
- Time lapse from assault
- Name of assailant (if known)
- Relationship of assailant to victim

History of assault
- Source of history
- Events preceding the assault
- Place of assault
- Drugs or alcohol consumed by the victim
- Details of the assault – to direct forensic sampling
- Damage or disruption to clothing
- Site and mechanism of injuries – to include details of any weapons or implements used
- Defence used by victim
- Any loss of consciousness

Exact nature of assault
- Digital/vaginal – Yes/No
- Oral/vaginal – Yes/No
- Oral/penile – Yes/No
- Penile/vaginal – Yes/No (If yes did ejaculation occur?)
- Penile/anal – Yes/No (If yes did ejaculation occur?)
- Digital/anal – Yes/No
- Lubricant or condom used?

Events following assault
- Changing of clothes
- Washing the genital area
- Taking a shower or bath
- Washing of hair
- Cleaning of teeth
- Micturition or defecation
- Vomiting
- Ingestion of food or drink
- Any medical treatment received since assault

Table 2. Relevant medical and sexual history

Gynaecological history
- Age at menarche
- LMP – forensic analysis cannot distinguish between menstrual blood and that related to injury
- Menstrual cycle
- Any gynaecological problems
  1. Current
  2. Past history

Obstetric history
- Pregnant – Presently/previously/never
- Outcome of previous pregnancies

Sexual history
- Sexually active? – Presently/previously/never
- Last coitus
  1. Date
  2. Time
  3. Use of lubricant? – Yes/No
- Genital problems – Past/present
- Sexually transmitted diseases – Yes/No

General medical history
- History of serious illness – Past/present
- Psychiatric problems – Yes/No
- Previous operations – Yes/No
- Bruising tendency – Yes/No
- Skin problems – Yes/No

Social history
- Current occupation

Table 3. Forensic samples to be taken at forensic medical examination

Non-intimate samples
- Control swabs – wet and dry
- Buccal swab – for DNA analysis if venesection refused
- Saliva specimen – if oral assault
- Skin swab – at site of kissing/sucking/ejaculation/bite (moistened if necessary)
- Head hair combings
- Head hair cuttings
- Right and left nail scrapings – if visible debris or if victim scratched assailant
- Nail cuttings – if broken nails or if victim scratched assailant
- Nail filings – to recover blood samples or skin fragments

Intimate samples
- Pubic hair combings
- Pubic hair cuttings
- Vulval swabs
- Introital swabs
- Low vaginal swabs
- Cervical swabs – should be taken if vaginal intercourse has taken place over 48 hours ago
- Anal and rectal swabs – a proctoscope may need to be used in cases of anal penetration
- High vaginal swabs – preferably four swabs should be taken
- Blood samples – for DNA analysis, blood typing, alcohol estimation, toxicology screen
- Tampon or sanitary towel – if used can be analysed for semen and body fluids
- Urine sample – for alcohol and toxicology testing
- Examination gown should be sent for analysis

CONSULT OTHER TOPICS
Domestic violence or abuse (p 36)
Emergency contraception (p 39)
Genital tract trauma (p 24)
Upper tract pelvic infection (p 13)
Vulval and lower tract genital infection (p 17)

SUPPLEMENTARY INFORMATION

Undertake a systematic forensic medical examination

Examination is often undertaken in 'rape suites' in police stations. A 'Sexual Offences Kit' should be used, which contains all the necessary equipment, such as swabs, gloves, disposable speculum, specimen bags and bottles, labels, scissors, combs, gown, a sheet of brown paper, information sheet and medical examination record. Assess emotional state, evidence of alcohol or drug intoxication, damage or staining to clothes, evidence of external injury. Clothing should be removed whilst standing on a sheet of brown paper and submitted for forensic examination. Document: (a) any injuries present that may relate to the incident on body charts and describe in detail; (b) relevant previous injuries; (c) any previous surgery or illness that may affect interpretation of the clinical findings.

Referral to the GUM Clinic for screening for STDs, HIV, and prophylaxis where indicated

Prophylaxis includes azithromycin/metronidazole +/− ciprofloxacin for STDs. Post-exposure prophylaxis for HIV, involves pre-HIV test counselling and informed consent. It should be offered to those with a negative baseline HIV ELISA test, if within 72 hours of the incident and is continued for 28 days. Offer vaccination against hepatitis and further treatment of any infections identified on screening for STDs. Follow-up at 3 months is arranged for syphilis, hepatitis and repeat HIV testing.

Completion of a 'professional witness' statement

This should include details of the history of the assault, relevant medical, surgical and psychiatric history, the normal and abnormal findings of the examination, the forensic specimens taken, any medical treatment given and post-examination arrangements made. The forensic medical examiner should give an opinion as to the degree of certainty about the likely cause of the injuries. The statement should have a professional appearance and be carefully checked for errors, prior to submission to the police. Any errors must be 'corrected' by preparing a supplementary statement. It must include a statutory declaration with the date and signature of the FME at the bottom of each page and at the end of the declaration. A witness should also sign each page. The FME should state their qualifications, appointment and relevant experience. New examining doctors should discuss the case and statement preparation with an experienced FME. Many police forces have standard statement forms that the FME completes.

Professionals involved should be aware of 'Rape Trauma Syndrome'

There is no typical reaction to rape. During the rape the victim may experience de-realization, de-personalization, disassociation, terror, confusion, helplessness and loss of physical control. Following the rape, symptoms of anxiety, depression, tear-fulness, flashbacks, humiliation, self-blame, disbelief, anger, fear, powerlessness, guilt, shame and physical revulsion are common. Long term problems with social adjustment, sexual relationships, physical health and substance abuse can occur.

FURTHER READING

Bamberger JD, Waldo CR, Gerberding JL et al. (1999) Post exposure prophylaxis for HIV infection following sexual assault. *Am. J. Med.* **106**: 323–326.

Bowyer L and Dalton ME (1997) Female victims of rape and their genital findings. *Br. J. Obstet. Gynaecol.* **104**: 617–620.

Cameron H (1997) Rape – including history and examination. In: Bewley S, Friend J and Mezey G (Eds) *Violence Against Women.* RCOG Press, London, pp. 245–261.

Cartwright PS and the Sexual Assault Study Group (1987) Factors that correlate with injury sustained by survivors of sexual assault. *Obstet. Gynecol.* **70**: 44–46.

Crane J (1996) Injury. In: McClay WDS (Ed.) *Clinical Forensic Medicine.* Greenwich Medical Media, London, pp. 143–162.

Gostin LO, Lazzarini, Z, Alexander D et al (1994) HIV testing, counselling and prophylaxis after sexual assault. *JAMA* **271**: 1436–1444.

Hampton HL (1995) Care of the woman who has been raped. *N. Engl. J. Med.* **332** (5): 234–237.

Holmes MM, Resnick HS, Kilpatrick DG and Best LB (1996) Rape-related pregnancy: estimated and descriptive characteristics from a national sample of women. *Am. J. Obstet. Gynecol.* **175**(2): 320–325.

Marchbanks PA, Liu KJ and Mercy JA (1990) Risk of injury from resisting rape. *Am. J. Epidemiol.* **132**: 540–549.

Mezey GC and Taylor PJ (1988) Psychological reactions of women who have been raped: A descriptive and comparative study. *Br. J. Psych.* **152:** 330–339.

Ramin SM, Satin AJ, Stone IC and Wendel GD (1992) Sexual assault in postmenopausal women. *Obstet. Gynecol.* **80:** 860–864.

Roberts R (1994) Rape crisis management. *Diplomate* **1**: 6–11.

Smugar SS, Spina BJ and Merz JF (2000) Informed consent for emergency contraception: variability in hospital care of rape victims. *Am. J. Public Health* **90(9):** 1372–1376.

Walch AG and Broadhead WE (1992) Prevalence of lifetime sexual victimisation among female patients. *J. Fam. Practice* **35**: 511–516.

Willott GM and Allard JE (1982) Spermatozoa – their persistence after sexual intercourse. *Forensic Sci. Int.* **19**: 135–154.

Willott GM and Crosse MM (1986) The detection of spermatozoa in the mouth. *J. Forensic Sci. Soc.* **26**: 125–128.

Wright AM, Duke L, Fraser E and Sviland L (1989) Northumbria women`s police doctor scheme: a new approach to examining victims of sexual assault. *BMJ* **298**: 1011–1012.

DOMESTIC VIOLENCE OR ABUSE

Helen Sullivan

Domestic abuse is physical, psychological, financial or sexual abuse by a partner or ex-partner. The overwhelming majority of victims are women. Domestic abuse is particularly relevant in obstetrics and gynaecology as it is a significant cause of gynaecological pathology and maternal and perinatal mortality and morbidity. Pregnancy may be a trigger for abuse to start. In 1998, the Royal College of Obstetricians and Gynaecologists estimated that a woman has a one in four chance of experiencing domestic abuse.

Suspect domestic abuse and remember that it has no cultural or class boundaries

The following groups are 'at risk':

- Women with pain problems.
- Women with multiple non-specific complaints.
- Women with unexplained injuries.
- Women who are divorced or separated.
- Women who abuse alcohol or drugs.
- Women who are poor attenders at out-patient clinics.
- Women who lack independent transport or access to a telephone.
- Women whose partners are 'over-involved'.
- Women who are reluctant or frightened to speak in front of their partner.
- Women where staff 'have a hunch'.

If domestic abuse is suspected

ACTION PLAN

To dig around use **'A SPADE'**

1 A 'Ask'
- Women do not mind being asked. Abused women want to be asked.

2 S 'Safely'
- Ask her away from her partner.
- Use professional authority to ask him to leave for a while.

3 P 'Privately'
- Do not ask her in front of the children or behind a curtain.
- Use independent interpreters if required.

4 A 'Attitude must be right'
- Be unhurried and non-judgmental.

5 D 'Direct questions'
- Ask direct questions that require a direct answer.

6 E 'Ear – listening'
- Hear what she is saying, requests for help are often veiled. She may try to 'test you out'.

Ask relevant questions

ACTION PLAN

1 **General**
- Is everything all right at home?
- Are you getting the support you need at home?

2 **Direct**
- I notice a number of bruises. How did they happen?
- Do you ever feel frightened of your partner?
- We all have rows at home sometimes. What happens when you and your partner disagree?
- Have you ever been in a relationship where you have been hit, punched or hurt in any way? Is this happening now?

When domestic abuse is admitted

ACTION PLAN

She has told you a 'SECRET'

1 **S Safety – is it safe for her to go home?**
- If not, discuss alternatives including requesting the local housing department to provide a place of safety, a women's refuge, friends, family or hospital admission.

2 **E Explore – her situation and feelings**
- 'Would you like to talk about what has happened to you?'
- 'What would you like to do about this?' This can in itself be therapeutic. Listen. Take her seriously. Take the view that abuse is not acceptable and may be illegal. Reinforce that she is not the problem and that it is not her fault.

3 **C Child protection**
- About half the men who abuse their partner pose an emotional or physical risk to their children. The best way to protect children is to support the non-abusing parent. Abused women have often been told by their partner that their children will be taken away from them as they are 'unfit'. Where you believe the children are at risk you have a duty to inform the local Child Protection Officer.
- Very rarely, it may be necessary to break the woman's confidence to protect her children. The General Medical Council advise that doctors 'should only break confidence when the relative costs and benefits of one individual's safety exceed another's right to privacy'. The GMC also states that it is essential to inform her *before* disclosure. Usually when a woman understands Social Services are extremely unlikely to remove the children from her care, she is happy to act in their best interests.

4 **R Records**
- Record with consent. She may not wish to take any action at the time of an assault but may agree a detailed record being kept confidential, in case she wishes to use it in the future. Record what she says happened. Record in detail what you find including non-bodily evidence like torn clothes. Body maps and photographs may be useful. DO NOT record any reference to domestic abuse in hand-held notes.

Domestic Violence or Abuse

- Discuss with her any plans for leaving. Suggest to her that she should leave when her partner is absent, as leaving can be dangerous. Suggest to her that she tries to collect some money, keys and essential documents for herself and her children.

6 **T Telephone numbers**

- Tell her telephone numbers of organizations that can help her in a crisis. You need your own list of local numbers. Ensure they are current. She may not be able to take written information with her but it may be helpful for her to know that the numbers are available in a particular place. The National Women's Aid Federation help-line number in 2001 is 08457 023468.
- DO NOT tell her that she must leave. It makes her feel misunderstood. Leaving is hard especially for a woman whose self-esteem has been damaged by abuse. Leaving is dangerous. It is the time of maximum danger for the woman. Leaving is difficult so she must make the decision herself. You may not see the effect of your intervention, which is frustrating but an appropriate response makes a positive contribution.

CONSULT OTHER TOPICS

Consent (p 279)
Genital tract trauma (p 24)
Management of the rape victim (p 30)

FURTHER READING

Bewley S, Friend J and Mazey G (eds) (1998) *Violence against women*. RCOG Press, London.
General Medical Council (2000) Confidentiality: protecting and providing information.
Royal College of Midwives (1997) *Domestic Abuse in Pregnancy*. Position paper.

EMERGENCY CONTRACEPTION

Niamh McCabe

Although 'Levonelle-2'® (progesterone-only post-coital contraception) is now available without medical prescription, many women still present to medical practitioners for emergency contraception. The commonest presentation is following unprotected intercourse or condom accident. However, emergency contraception may also be indicated if combined oral contraceptive pills (COCP) or progesterone only pills (POP) have been missed, if a 'DepoProvera' injection is not given within 89 days of the previous one, if a diaphragm has been incorrectly used or an IUCD is removed mid-cycle.

The risk of pregnancy varies greatly depending mainly on the timing of intercourse in the menstrual cycle. It is also affected by the woman's age. As modern hormonal emergency contraception is relatively safe, it is better to err on the side of caution and treat a woman who presents even if the risk of pregnancy is low.

ACTION PLAN

1 **Assess risk of conception**

2 **Consider contra-indications**

3 **Ascertain and discuss options**

3a. **MINI ACTION PLAN – Hormonal contraception**
- Prescribe 'Levonelle-2'® 0.75 mg tablets.
- One to be taken as soon as possible after intercourse.
- Repeat 12 hours later.

3b. **MINI ACTION PLAN – IUCD insertion**
- Administer azithromycin 1 g and metronidazole 2 g po.
- Lithotomy: perform VE to ascertain uterine size and attitude.
- Pass Cusco`s speculum.
- Take HVS and endocervical swab for chlamydia.
- Clean cervix with chlorhexidine.
- Administer local anaesthetic (3% prilocaine with felypressin, 'Citanest with Octapressin`®) using a dental syringe – insert needle at least 2 cm into cervix at 2, 4, 8 and 10 o`clock).
- Grasp anterior lip of cervix with single-toothed tenaculum or vulsellum.
- Pass uterine sound to assess length of cavity.
- Prepare and insert IUCD according to manufacturer`s instructions.
- Trim threads.
- Gently pass sterile sound to ensure end of IUCD is not within cervical canal.
- Prescribe diclofenac 50 mg tds for 1–2 days.

4 **Arrange ongoing contraception**

5 **Arrange follow-up**
- Advise further review if next menses is >7 days late.

CONSULT OTHER TOPICS

Complications of the intrauterine contraceptive device (p 42)
Pregnancy with an intrauterine contraceptive device present (p 107)

SUPPLEMENTARY INFORMATION

Assess risk of conception

Determine length of cycle, date of LMP and timing of first act of unprotected sexual intercourse (SI). Risk of conception in peri-ovulatory days is 20–30% if no contraception is used. Count hours since SI. Emergency contraception should be advised if:

- no contraception or condom accident;
- COCP – missed pill:
  - a two or more missed pills from first 7 pills in any combination;
  - b two or more missed pills from last 7 pills in any combination (unless new packet started immediately);
  - c four or more missed pills in any combination mid-packet.

  Note: 1 day on antibiotics = '1 missed pill'
- POP – missed pill: at risk for 7 days after pill missed or if pill taken more than 3 hours late.
- 'DepoProvera': at risk if intercourse occurs more than day 89 from last injection.
- IUCD: at risk if IUCD removed on day 7–17 and intercourse occurred in previous 7 days.

Consider contra-indications

Pregnancy is the only true contraindication to progesterone-only emergency contraception. Pregnancy test/pelvic exam is not routinely indicated but have a high index of suspicion for possibility of pregnancy. Current or past history of PID precludes insertion of an IUCD as emergency contraception.

Ascertain options

- <72 hours since first act of intercourse = 'Levonelle-2'® or IUCD.
- >72 hours but within 5 days of calculated day of ovulation = IUCD.

'Levonelle-2'®

The progesterone-only medication, 'Levonelle-2'® is now the preferred hormonal method of emergency contraception as it is more effective and has less side-effects than the combined oestrogen and progesterone emergency contraceptive 'PC4'®. It is packaged as two tablets, each containing 0.75 mg of levonorgestrel. It causes less vomiting than 'PC4'®, but women should be advised that if vomiting occurs within 3 hours of taking the tablet, the second should be taken straight away and arrangements made to obtain a further tablet. The efficacy of 'Levonelle-2'® is not affected by broad-spectrum antibiotics (e.g. ampicillin, tetracycline) but enzyme-inducing drugs such as anti-epileptic and anti-tuberculous medications do render it less effective. In this situation, increase the dose by 50% (i.e. two tablets followed by one tablet 12 hours later).

Emergency Contraception

Copper IUCD

A copper-bearing IUCD may be used and is more effective than hormonal emergency contraception. However, it is not usually as widely available as hormonal methods. It can be uncomfortable to insert in nulliparous women, and carries a small risk of causing pelvic infection. If inserting an IUCD as an emergency, swabs should be taken to allow contact tracing, but prophylactic antibiotics should be given anyway.

Arrange ongoing contraception

Following 'Levonelle-2'® use

If no contraception has been used, advise abstinence until next menses. Advise starting a reliable contraceptive on day 1 of menses if still sexually active (e.g. the COCP).

If used because of 'missed pills', advise omitting pills on the day of emergency contraception but continue with rest of packet. Use barrier method until 7 consecutive pills taken. If 'DepoProvera` was late by <5 days, give next 'DepoProvera` and advise barrier method for next 7 days.

Following IUCD insertion

IUCD can be left in as ongoing contraception. Failure rate is 0.4–2.4 per 100 woman years. If the woman subsequently wishes removal of the IUCD, remove at the time of menstruation and commence another reliable contraceptive such as the COCP.

Follow-up

Routine follow-up is not necessary. Review should be arranged if the next period is more than 7 days late, or it is very light.

If a sexually transmitted disease is detected, follow-up at a GUM clinic should be arranged.

If an IUCD has been inserted, follow-up for removal with menses should be arranged (unless it is to be used for ongoing contraception).

FURTHER READING

Faculty of Family Planning and Reproductive Health Care, Royal College of Obstetricians and Gynaecologists Guidance (2000) Emergency contraception: recommendations for clinical practice. *Br. J. Fam. Plan.* **26**(2): 93–96.

COMPLICATIONS OF THE INTRAUTERINE CONTRACEPTIVE DEVICE

Niamh McCabe and Kim Hinshaw

The IUCD is a very reliable form of reversible contraception but there are some specific problems which can present on an emergency basis. The majority of IUCDs used at the present time in the UK are copper-based. An increasing number of women are using the levonorgesterol intrauterine system (LNG-IUS 'Mirena'®). This progesterone-coated IUCD is popular because of its increased efficacy and improved side-effect profile. It is important to remember that with several complications related to IUCD use, contraceptive efficacy is reduced or lost. The woman may already be pregnant or be in need of additional contraception when she presents.

The common complications are:

- Lost threads.
- Perforation – complete or partial.
- Infection.
- Pregnancy – intrauterine or ectopic.
- Menorrhagia.

Less common is:

- Translocation (spontaneous migration via the uterine wall) – incidence 0.2%.

CONSULT OTHER TOPICS

Ectopic pregnancy (p 76)
Emergency contraception (p 39)
Pregnancy with an intrauterine contraceptive device present (p 107)
Upper tract pelvic infection (p 13)

LOST THREADS

1 **Check pregnancy test**

2 **Perform speculum +/– digital vaginal examination**
- The woman may simply be unused to feeling the threads.
- Confirm if threads are visible.
- Confirm that IUCD is not visible within external cervical os or canal.

3 **If threads not visible attempt to bring them into view**
- Pass a sterile Spencer-Wells forceps into the cervical canal.
- Use an 'Emmett' IUCD-thread retriever.
- Use a cylindrical nylon brush (as used for taking endocervical smears).

4 **If unsuccessful – arrange an ultrasound scan**

5 **IUCD in the uterine cavity on scan**
- If IUCD in 'incorrect position' (i.e. low in uterine cavity) – consider removal and replacement as contraceptive efficacy may be reduced.

- If IUCD in correct position – patient will not be able to reassure herself about retention of the device by self-examination. Consider replacement. Alternatively – offer ultrasound check annually.

6 **IUCD not in the uterine cavity on scan**
- Expulsion is the most likely diagnosis.
- If patient is unaware of expulsion, consider translocation or perforation.

7 **Consider immediate contraceptive needs**

8 **Management if pregnant**
- Consider site of pregnancy.
- Is IUCD in the uterus?

SUPPLEMENTARY INFORMATION

If threads not visible attempt to bring them into view

The Emmett-IUCD thread retriever is a hook-like instrument with multiple notches which is passed into the uterus and used like a curette to try and trap the threads. It is disposable but its use may require analgesia and/or local anaesthesia. A small nylon brush, such as the 'Cytobrush'®, may be gently rotated within the cervical canal, trapping the thread in the bristles and aiding retrieval.

If unsuccessful – arrange an ultrasound scan

The LNG-IUS is more difficult to see on ultrasound as echo returns are less defined than those from copper-based devices. Clearly document on the request form the type of IUCD.

IUCD not in the uterine cavity on scan

In this situation, consider whether expulsion, complete perforation or translocation has occurred. Expulsion occurs in 1–7% of cases in the first year of use (most commonly in the first 3 months). Abdominal/pelvic X-ray is mandatory if complete perforation or translocation is suspected and ultrasound does not detect the device. Only diagnose expulsion if the patient is sure that she can definitely confirm seeing the device. Remember that a translocated IUCD may be anywhere in the peritoneal cavity. An X-ray must therefore include both diaphragms.

Consider immediate contraceptive needs

Offer emergency oral contraception ('Levonelle-2'®) if IUCD expulsion is within 7 days and 'unprotected' intercourse has occurred. Otherwise, exclude pregnancy and arrange alternative long-term contraception.

Management if pregnant

In pregnancy, the threads may be 'lost' because the uterus is enlarging, drawing the threads into the cervical canal. If the pregnancy test is positive, urgent ultrasound examination is necessary to exclude ectopic pregnancy and to confirm whether the IUCD is still in the uterus. Specific management when pregnancy occurs with an IUCD *in situ* is discussed in another chapter.

PERFORATION

Most commonly occurs at the time of insertion (estimated incidence 1.3 per 1000 insertions). It may be recognized by an experienced operator. It is commoner if a tenaculum is not used to apply counter-traction to the cervix to correct ante or retroversion.

ACTION PLAN

1 **Early presentation – perforation suspected at time of insertion**
   - Attempt removal by applying gentle traction on the threads (this may be successful with partial perforation).
   - If unsuccessful and no further pain – arrange urgent ultrasound scan.
   - Continuing severe pain – refer for emergency gynaecological opinion.

2 **Late presentation – may present as 'lost' thread or with pregnancy**

3 **If IUCD is not in uterus, expulsion is the likely reason, HOWEVER**
   - Perforation must be excluded if patient cannot confirm expulsion.

4 **Arrange ultrasound to confirm position of IUCD**

5 **Late presentation with partial perforation – attempt removal by gentle traction**

6 **Laparoscopy or laparotomy**
   - Consent for laparoscopic retrieval of IUCD.
   - Consent for possible laparotomy.

SUPPLEMENTARY INFORMATION

Arrange ultrasound to confirm position of IUCD

The radiographer should be informed that perforation is suspected. Careful scan assessment in two planes, can diagnose partial perforation. It cannot reliably confirm complete perforation as the device may be in the upper abdomen and outwith the range of the transducer. Bowel gas may also obscure an IUCD at scan.

Late presentation with partial perforation

Again, grasp the thread or visible end of the IUCD and apply GENTLE traction. Stop if there is any resistance, as partial perforation may be associated with bladder or bowel adhesions.

Laparoscopy or laparotomy

If the perforation is recent the device is usually visible and accessible at laparoscopy as adhesion formation should be minimal. Laparoscopic removal should be possible. If it is embedded in adhesions, the bladder wall, bowel wall or mesentery, a laparotomy will be required. It may be appropriate to involve a colorectal surgeon or urologist if the device has penetrated the bowel or bladder. If there is a delay in performing the laparoscopy, the woman should be advised to report urgently any abdominal pain, particularly if associated with bladder or bowel disturbance.

INFECTION

The risk of infection is only increased above the background risk for the first 30 days after insertion. After this the risk is related to the demographic profile of the woman (i.e. age, number of sexual partners, etc.)

1 **Check pregnancy test**

2 **Take HVS for C&S, and endocervical (+/– urethral) swabs for *Chlamydia* and *Gonococcus***

3 **If clinically mild disease – leave IUCD *in situ*.** Treat with:
- Doxycycline 200 mg stat followed by 100 mg daily for 14 days.
- Metronidazole 400 mg tds for 5 days.

4 **Analgesia**
- NSAIDs are effective.

5 **Consider IUCD removal**
- If severe constitutional upset.
- If no improvement after 48 hours of treatment.
- If pelvic abscess suspected.

6 **Referral to GUM for contact tracing if indicated**

SUPPLEMENTARY INFORMATION

Check pregnancy test

The symptoms of upper tract pelvic infection are similar to EP.

Consider IUCD removal

A lower threshold for removal may be appropriate in nulliparous women because of the risk of tubal infertility. Remember to give emergency hormonal contraception if there has been intercourse in the preceding 7 days. The management of pelvic abscess is discussed elsewhere.

PREGNANCY

Always consider pregnancy in any woman fitted with an IUCD who presents with lost threads, abnormal bleeding or pain. Copper-based devices reduce the overall risk of pregnancy by 80% compared to 'no contraceptive use'. The LNG-IUS reduces the risk by 90%. The management of ectopic pregnancy and intrauterine pregnancy with an IUCD *in situ* are fully discussed in other chapters.

MENORRHAGIA

Copper-based IUCDs cause increased prostaglandin release in the endometrium and increase menstrual blood loss by around 50% on average. Fifteen percent of women will have the IUCD removed because of this side effect. This action plan reviews management of heavy bleeding in association with the copper IUCD.

ACTION PLAN

1 **Exclude pregnancy complications – miscarriage and EP**

2 **Pelvic examination**
- Check threads.
- Look for other pathology such as fibroids.
- Take swabs to exclude pelvic infection.

3 **Ultrasound and endometrial sampling if over 40**

4 **First-line treatment**
- Tranexamic acid 1 g qds and mefenamic acid 500 mg tds.

5 **Consider removal and replacement with LNG-IUS if no response to above treatment**

FURTHER READING

Ben-Rafael Z and Bider D (1996) A new procedure for removal of a lost intrauterine device. *Obstet. Gynecol.* **87(5):** 785–786.

Complications of the IUCD

CHILDHOOD EMERGENCIES

Niamh McCabe and Kim Hinshaw

Minor trauma and retained foreign bodies are the commonest emergency paediatric problems in gynaecology. Careful history and sensitive examination are crucial because of the immaturity and natural embarrassment of the patient. It is important to have a high index of suspicion for sexual abuse and if it is suspected a senior paediatric opinion should be sought. Gynaecology trainees should discuss the case with the consultant before undertaking an examination. Ideally, the girl should be examined by one senior doctor in order to keep distress to a minimum. It will also reduce the risk of forensic evidence being lost.

CONSIDER OTHER TOPICS

Consent (p 279)
Genital tract trauma (p 24)
Toxic shock syndrome (p 22)
Vulval and lower tract genital infection (p 17)

RETAINED FOREIGN BODY

The patient is usually a toddler, but may be an intellectually impaired older girl. In toddlers, the object is often a small toy. Presentation may be with vaginal discharge or bleeding noticed by the mother. Tampons are often retained in teenagers who have recently started menstruation. Presentation is usually with a foul-smelling vaginal discharge or irregular bleeding. Rarely, it may present with Toxic Shock Syndrome. Objects may be retained when used for masturbation. The young woman will be acutely embarrassed. The history may be obtained best by female nursing staff.

ACTION PLAN

1 **Obtain appropriate parental consent prior to examination**

2 **Consider possibility of sexual assault**

3 **Pelvic examination**
- Including inspection of perianal region, vulva and introitus as well as insertion of vaginal speculum.

4 **Record findings**

5 **Take swabs for microbiology**

6 **Removal**
- Tampons and small objects may be removed with sponge-holding or polyp forceps. Larger objects may become impacted and require removal under anaesthesia.

SUPPLEMENTARY INFORMATION

Pelvic examination

In very young or mentally handicapped girls it will not be possible to examine in the clinic or ward. Indeed, vulval inspection may be declined. Consent should be obtained from the legal guardian and an examination performed under general anaesthesia.

In young children, a disrupted hymen is strongly suggestive of sexual assault.

Take swabs for microbiology

Antibiotic treatment is not usually necessary once the foreign body has been removed but any evidence of sexually transmitted infection will require urgent paediatric referral for assessment. Other support agencies may then become involved (e.g. hospital social work department).

Removal

The following regimen or something similar, should be used when removing a foreign body under GA.

- Examine the patient in lithotomy.
- If the child is young, consider examination with a small nasal speculum (obtained from the ENT department) or alternatively an otoscope. This will probably leave the hymen intact.
- Liberally lubricate the foreign body – this alone may be sufficient to allow its removal.
- Grasp the edge of the object with sponge forceps and apply gentle traction. Certain objects (such as the tops of deodorant sprays) may need to be turned round within the vagina in order to grasp an edge.
- Consider careful crushing/reduction of the foreign body if this can be achieved without vaginal trauma.
- Check the vagina for lacerations.

VAGINAL DISCHARGE

This is a very worrying symptom for most parents because of the spectre of sexual abuse. It is usually benign and easily managed but if abuse is suspected, an appropriate referral should be made. Again with young children, adequate examination may only be possible in theatre.

ACTION PLAN

1 **Brief history of the nature of the discharge**
- A white-yellow discharge is normal in prepubertal girls and simple education and reassurance may be all that is required.
- A blood-stained discharge may be the first signs of menstruation. The age of puberty is falling. Look for signs of breast development etc.

2 **Inspection of the vulva**
- Look for evidence of scratching, discharge, trauma.

3 **Swabs**
- Consider need to swab for *Chlamydia* and *Gonococcus*.
- Swab for *Candida* – consider diabetes.

4 **If a foreign body is suspected, manage as above**

5 **Treat with antibiotics as appropriate**
- Vaginal infection in prepubertal girls is usually due to *Streptococci* and responds to oral penicillin V.

SUPPLEMENTARY INFORMATION

Brief history of the nature of the discharge

A foul-smelling discharge suggests a foreign body. In the presence of a persistent blood-stained discharge, rare malignancies such as 'sarcoma botyroides' should be considered. Is there any evidence of precocious puberty? Isolated pruritus may suggest infestation with the very common threadworm.

VULVOVAGINITIS/LABIAL FUSION

This is fairly common in childhood and usually presents with vulval soreness +/– dyspareunia. Presentation may be acute with severe excoriation and pain. It is often due to over or under-zealous vulval hygiene. Discuss vulval hygiene with the parents. Repeated courses of antibiotics may have disrupted the normal flora – consider candidiasis. The various causes of dermatitis should also be considered.

ACTION PLAN

1 **Inspect the vulva**
- Soreness and redness are common.

2 **Take swabs (consider exclusion of STDs)**

3 **Check MSU**
- Check for glycosuria and exclude infection.
- Consider enuresis – barrier cream if confirmed.

4 **Consider the 'sellotape' test if threadworms are suspected**

5 **Consider 'dermatitis'**
- Chemical (enuresis).
- Atopic (does child have eczema?).
- Lichen sclerosis (associated with fissuring).

6 **Advise re: gentle washing (from front to back)**
- Avoidance of bubble baths, cosmetics etc.

7 **Consider short-term use of local oestrogen cream**

SUPPLEMENTARY INFORMATION

Inspect the vulva

Bear sexual abuse in mind and refer on if suspicious.

Consider the 'Sellotape' test if threadworms are suspected

A piece of sellotape is applied to the peri-anal skin to trap the eggs of worms as they come out to lay at night. Treatment is with rigorous handwashing after toileting, wearing tight underclothes at night to prevent peri-anal scratching and propagation of the infection. The whole family should be treated with mebendazole 200 mg (except for children under 2 years of age).

Consider 'dermatitis'

Atopic dermatitis may affect the vulva – refer to dermatologist. Lichen sclerosis can affect prepubertal girls but resolves at puberty. Severe itching, atrophy and fissuring require treatment with short-term local oestrogen. Lichen sclerosis is associated with labial fusion. If asymptomatic, no intervention required. If treatment is required:

- local oestrogen cream for 2–3 weeks;
- majority will separate spontaneously;
- bland barrier cream/petroleum jelly to prevent re-fusion.

IMPERFORATE HYMEN ('HAEMATOCOLPOS')

Although this is the commonest congenital abnormality of the female genital tract it is still rare. It usually presents in teenage girls aged 14–15 years with a history of cyclical lower abdominal pain for several months and primary amenorrhea. A mass is palpable in the lower abdomen and the intact hymen is distended, often with a bluish hue. The distended vagina is full of blood and the mass can be felt bimanually on rectal examination. Rarely, haematocolpos can present with acute urinary retention.

ACTION PLAN

1 **Discuss diagnosis and management with family**

2 **Arrange examination under anaesthesia**

3 **Lithotomy position**

4 **Make cruciate incision in the hymen**
- AP and tranverse incisions.
- Sutures are not usually required.
- No need to excise hymenal remnants – healing is excellent.
- Local infiltration with 0.5% bupivacaine for post-operative pain.

5 **Allow accumulated menses to drain**
- Will have a heavy brown, red loss for several days.
- Thereafter onset of normal menstruation.

6 **Long-term follow-up is not necessary, but the girl and her family should be reassured. If menstruation becomes regular, there are no long-term sequelae in terms of future fertility**

PERINEAL/VULVAL TRAUMA

In young children, the commonest cause of perineal trauma is accidental straddle injury. Parents are particularly distressed as there may be direct vulval trauma with compression tears of the labia or fourchette, or a vulval haematoma. In most cases if bleeding has settled and the external vulva can be visualized, routine suturing is not required. If there is any doubt as to the extent of injury, if bleeding continues or if tissue is obviously misaligned, an examination under anaesthetic should be arranged.

An action plan for the management of this problem is discussed in the chapter 'Genital tract trauma'.

FURTHER READING

Edmonds DK (1999) Gynaecological disorders of childhood and adolescence. In: Edmonds DK (Ed) *Dewhurst`s Textbook of Obstetrics and Gynaecology for Postgraduates,* 6th edn. Blackwell Science, Oxford, pp. 12–16.

GYNAECOLOGICAL EMERGENCIES IN THE OLDER WOMAN

Niamh McCabe and Kim Hinshaw

Acute gynaecology in older women is often complicated by co-existent chronic medical conditions. Early involvement of the anaesthetist is recommended if surgical treatment is planned. Malignant disease is also commoner in the older age group so one must maintain a high index of suspicion for underlying malignancies. Although older women may suffer from many of the same acute gynaecological conditions as younger women, the following conditions are much commoner in the older population:

- Pyometra.
- Acute retention of urine.
- Incarcerated pessary.
- Irreducible prolapse.
- Significant post-menopausal bleeding.

CONSULT OTHER TOPICS

Acute abdominal pain (p 1)
Non-pregnant causes of vaginal bleeding (p 59)
Septic shock (p 267)
Surgical management of ovarian cysts in the pregnant and non-pregnant (p 6)
Unsuspected gynaecological malignancy (p 201)
Urinary tract infection (p 265)
Emergency presentations associated with prolapse (p 159)

PYOMETRA

Although pyometra may be an incidental finding at the time of hysteroscopy, presentation can be acute with a history of pelvic pain, general malaise and pyrexia. Often there is little or no vaginal loss. There may be a light, intermittent purulent discharge with a small amount of vaginal bleeding. The patient may present several days after undergoing outpatient endometrial biopsy. There is an association with underlying malignancy (usually endometrial) which will need to be excluded with appropriate investigation.

ACTION PLAN

1 **Admit**
   - Women with pyometra are often unwell, with varying degrees of pelvic pain.
   - There may be intermittent high fever and the enlarged uterus is usually exquisitely tender on bimanual examination.

2 **FBC, U&Es, random glucose. Endocervical and vaginal swabs, blood cultures**
   - The white cell count is raised. Vaginal discharge is not invariably present but swabs should be taken.

- Temperature >38°C may indicate bacteraemia and blood cultures should be taken.

3 **iv access and antibiotics**

4 **Analgesia**
- Opiate analgesia may be necessary.

5 **Pelvic ultrasound**

6 **Cervical dilatation under GA**
- Care with uterine sound – avoid perforation.
- Dilate cervix to at least 8 mm if possible.

7 **Interval hysteroscopy (minimum interval 7 days)**

8 **Endometrial/cervical malignancy excluded – arrange outpatient follow-up**

SUPPLEMENTARY INFORMATION

IV access and antibiotics

Pyometra is usually caused by a mixed infection with aerobic and anaerobic bacteria. 'Co-amoxiclav' or a third-generation cephalosporin have good activity against both but metronidazole may be added in severe infection. If the patient is toxic, discuss case with a consultant microbiologist. Consider triple antibiotic therapy (including gentamicin) with appropriate monitoring of renal function.

Pelvic ultrasound

Both TA and TV approaches may be necessary. Be aware that older women will be more concerned about the use of the TV route. Ultrasound will confirm fluid in a distended endometrial cavity. The real purpose of scanning is to exclude a foreign body such as a forgotten IUCD. It is unlikely that any useful information will be obtained regarding the presence, or otherwise, of an underlying carcinoma. The echo returns of pus show mixed heterogeneous shadowing which will obscure detail.

Cervical dilatation under GA

Instrumentation of the uterus should not be undertaken until at least 24–48 hours after antibiotics are started and preferably when signs of systemic illness are settling. GA is required to allow adequate drainage. Regional anaesthesia may be appropriate if there are underlying medical problems, but should be used cautiously in the presence of bacteraemia. The case should be discussed with senior anaesthetic staff. The cervix should be dilated to between 8 and 10 mm if possible. Care should be taken on inserting the uterine sound as perforation is more likely.

Interval hysteroscopy

This is necessary to exclude underlying endometrial malignancy but must be delayed, as adequate visualization of the endometrium is impossible in the presence of a pyometra. If the patient's general health is extremely poor, hysteroscopy may be done under local anaesthesia if necessary. In that situation, repeat TV scan with outpatient endometrial biopsy could also be considered as an interval procedure.

Endometrial/cervical malignancy excluded

The patient should be followed up to ensure that symptoms do not return. Recurrent symptoms may require definitive treatment in the form of hysterectomy.

ACUTE RETENTION OF URINE

Acute retention of urine can occur at any age but is more common in older women. It may be caused by constipation, drugs such as anticholinergics, surgery or pelvic masses. Unless the cause is obvious (i.e. an acute urinary tract infection) it is important to exclude an underlying mass and in particular, malignancy.

ACTION PLAN

1 **Confirm retention of urine**

2 **Pass Foley catheter**

3 **Send urine for urgent microscopy; culture and sensitivity**
- Treat pre-existing infection with appropriate antibiotics.

4 **Reassess: abdominal, pelvic and neurological examination**
- Exclude underlying obstructive mass.
- Exclude underlying acute neurological cause.

5 **Mass suspected – arrange pelvic ultrasound**

6 **Allow bladder to drain for at least 48 hours**
- Continuous drainage – no advantage in clamping and releasing 4 hourly.
- Record fluid balance.

7 **Remove catheter: measure voided volumes; check residual volumes (consider ultrasound)**

8 **Review: medications/bowel habit/mobility**

9 **If retention recurs – consider suprapubic catheter (SPC)**

10 **Consider urodynamics – if retention recurs and no cause found**

11 **Seek specialist help**
- Urological opinion.
- Specialist nurse.

12 **Long-term management: may require clean intermittent self-catheterization (CISC), SPC, urinary diversion**

SUPPLEMENTARY INFORMATION

Pass Foley catheter

An urethral Foley catheter size 12–14F is usually considered first (French gauge is equivalent to the circumference in millimetres) with SPC reserved for those with recurrent acute episodes of retention.

Reassess: abdominal, pelvic and neurological examination

A repeat pelvic examination should be performed after catheterization to check for pelvic masses. Assess for neurological deficit – in particular, check the 'saddle' distribution (S2,3,4) for any sensory loss.

Mass suspected – arrange pelvic ultrasound

Ovarian masses and large fibroids are the commonest masses causing acute retention in older women. If an ovarian mass is detected, CA125 should be checked and the woman referred to a gynaecological oncologist if necessary. Hysterectomy is required if fibroids are causing retention.

Allow bladder to drain for at least 48 hours

Free drainage must be continued for at least 48 hours. If the residual volume is significantly >1000 ml, it may be left for 5–7 days. Outpatient management may be appropriate at this stage. May need continued drainage until underlying cause is treated (e.g. large pelvic mass).

Remove catheter

Trial without catheter requires admission unless close liaison can be arranged in the community with a nurse specialist. The catheter is removed and all voided urine is measured. Volume of adequate voids should be over 250 ml. If the woman is unable to pass urine, consider a further attempt with a urethral catheter. Thereafter a SPC may be required and can be inserted under local anaesthetic.

Residual volumes may be measured using an 'in & out' disposable catheter. However, this will increase the risk of UTI and ideally residual volume can be rapidly and accurately assessed using a small portable ultrasound machine. Residual volume immediately post-void should be less than 150 ml.

Review medications/bowel habit/mobility

In the elderly, polypharmacy is common and medications should be reviewed. Ensure mobility and access to toileting are adequate. Treat severe constipation aggressively before catheter removal.

Consider urodynamics

Acute retention in the absence of an obstructing mass, may be due to bladder hypocontractility or urethral obstruction/stricture. Urodynamic assessment is helpful in differentiating these conditions. Urethral stricture responds to dilatation while bladder hypocontractility will require clean intermittent self-catheterisation (CISC). CISC is easily taught and most patients can manage this themselves. It may be required 2–3 times daily on average.

INCARCERATED PESSARY

Ring or shelf pessaries are used to control uterovaginal prolapse in women who are unfit for or reluctant to have definitive surgery. Modern devices are made of inert plastic and may be safely left *in situ* for up to 12 months. If left longer than this they may become epithelialized and require removal under anaesthesia, or they may cause severe ulceration and infection. Occasionally, pessaries *in situ* for a shorter time may also be difficult to remove, particularly if the woman's weight has changed markedly or when an inappropriate size of pessary has been inserted.

1 **Perform VE and attempt to remove pessary**
   - Ring pessary – hook index finger over the front and compress pessary from side to side with the thumb and middle finger as it is withdrawn.
   - Shelf pessaries – hook index finger over the pessary indentation anteriorly. Slide finger laterally, break the 'suction' effect and depress it to dislodge the pessary. Ensure handle is not forced into the vaginal wall but is guided down the vagina and passes out of introitus.

2 **If unsuccessful, take swabs for C&S and prescribe local oestrogen for 2 weeks then re-try**

3 **If still unsuccessful, assess mobility of pessary within the vagina**

4 **Removal under anaesthesia – may be necessary if deemed essential clinically or the pessary has become epithelialized**

5 **Consider topical oestrogen cream for 1 month to encourage healing**

6 **Review suitability for definitive surgery**

SUPPLEMENTARY INFORMATION

Perform VE and try to remove pessary

If the pessary is freely mobile and a finger can be passed all the way around it, removal is not essential. Repeated checks of mobility may be made every 6 months. Ensure integrity of vaginal mucosa is maintained – suspect trauma if bleeding or persistent discharge develops.

Removal under anaesthesia

Pessaries tend to be used in older, more infirm women, so early involvement of the anaesthetist to assess the most suitable mode of anaesthesia is essential. Once anaesthesia is established, the manoeuvres as described above are repeated. If the pessary has epithelialized, the overlying skin is incised and the pessary removed. This can be achieved with needle diathermy using an appropriate blend setting (cut/coagulate).

IRREDUCIBLE PROLAPSE

The prolapse will usually be a procidentia which has been neglected and become oedematous, ulcerated and infected. Pain may be a significant presenting symptom or alternatively, urinary retention.

1 **Admit**

2 **Catheterize if necessary (may need SPC)**

3 **Swab the prolapsed uterus for C&S**
- Treat infection as necessary.

4 **Check U&Es**
- The ureters may be kinked by the prolapse and cause renal impairment due to obstruction.

5 **Gentle attempt at replacement in vagina**
- Pack the vagina with oestrogen-imbued packs for 1–2 weeks.
- Healing is usually rapid once prolapse is reduced.

6 **If vaginal replacement is unsuccessful – apply topical oestrogen twice daily with betadine soaks if heavily infected. Replace within vagina when swelling settles**

7 **Consider replacement under GA if necessary (manage as per step 5)**

8 **Insert pessary to control or arrange for definitive surgery**

POST-MENOPAUSAL BLEEDING

This is defined as any bleeding from the genital tract more than 12 months after the last menstrual period. The average age of the menopause is rising and is presently 52 years. The older the woman, the more the likelihood of finding an underlying malignancy. Light to moderate bleeding may be investigated on an urgent outpatient basis but heavy bleeding will often require emergency admission.

1 **Admit**

2 **Assess degree of bleeding – institute resuscitation if required**

3 **Establish iv access – send blood for FBC, group and save**
- X-match and coagulation screen as clinically indicated.

4 **Review history of bleeding episode**
- Duration, amount, association with abdominal pain, associated discharge.

5 **Obtain MSU – exclude gross haematuria. Arrange microscopy, C&S**

6 **Abdominal examination – exclude a palpable mass**

7 **Pelvic examination**
- Exclude severe atrophic vaginitis – visualize the vaginal walls.
- Exclude vascular urethral caruncle or haematuria.
- See and feel the cervix – consider vascular polyp/carcinoma.
- Confirm uterine size and exclude adnexal mass.
- Consider trauma or assault (rare).

8 **Acute management – depends on underlying cause**
- Consider blood transfusion.

- Vaginal packing may be needed to control heavy local bleeding.
- Rarely, bleeding will need to be controlled in theatre under anaesthetic.

9 **Arrange further investigation**

10 **Involve appropriate specialists**

SUPPLEMENTARY INFORMATION

Obtain MSU – exclude gross haematuria

The source of bleeding is not always obvious to the patient. A careful history may suggest the possibility of gross haematuria or even rectal bleeding. Ask nursing staff to observe for either of these if you suspect bleeding is not gynaecological in origin.

Pelvic examination

An urethral caruncle is common in elderly females. It looks like a 'raspberry'-like, pedunculated granulomatous lesion attached to the posterior urethra near the external meatus. It is approximately the size of a 'pea' and consists of highly vascular connective tissue.

Acute management

Heavy bleeding related to a vascular lesion in the vagina (e.g. vascular polyp, carcinoma) may need temporary packing. The pack should be lubricated (e.g. 'Proflavine'). It should be inserted with care, but needs to be firm enough to apply local pressure to the bleeding area. A Sim's speculum and long packing forceps are ideal. If the vagina is packed appropriately, voiding will be compromised and the bladder should be drained using a Foley catheter.

If bleeding is intractable (as may be the case with gross cervical malignancy) control may only be obtained in theatre under general anaesthesia. Consider involvement of interventional radiologist and arterial embolization.

Arrange further investigation

- Suspected carcinoma – arrange appropriate biopsy (endometrial, cervical, vulval).
- Ultrasound scan.
- Formal EUA hysteroscopy and endometrial biopsy may be required.
- Referral to gynaecological oncologist – for formal staging or definitive treatment.

NON-PREGNANT CAUSES OF VAGINAL BLEEDING

Niamh McCabe and Kim Hinshaw

Heavy vaginal bleeding can occur at any age and may present as an acute emergency. Complications of pregnancy should always be considered and excluded. This may be the first presenting symptom of malignancy. The main action plan below reviews the general approach to emergency management of heavy vaginal bleeding. Thereafter, mini-action plans are given describing management of some specific problems which are not covered in other parts of this book.

Non-pregnant causes of heavy vaginal bleeding:

- Severe dysfunctional uterine bleeding/menorrhagia.
- Cervical polyps/fibroid polyps.
- Secondary haemorrhage after major gynaecological surgery.
- Genital tract trauma (including rape).
- Bleeding post LLETZ or cone biopsy.
- Bleeding due to malignancy (vulval, vaginal, cervical, uterine).
- Post-menopausal bleeding.

CONSULT OTHER TOPICS

Hysterectomy (p 128)
Genital tract trauma (p 24)
Gynaecological emergencies in the older woman (p 52)
Haemorrhage control (p 197)
Management of the rape victim (p 30)

Emergency management of heavy vaginal bleeding (non-pregnant)

ACTION PLAN

1 **Resuscitate as indicated – follow ABCs. Establish venous access**

2 **Take brief history**
- LMP, duration of bleeding, recent surgery/trauma/abnormal smear.

3 **General examination**
- Pulse, BP, pallor, bruising.

4 **Abdominal examination**
- Look for masses, tenderness.

5 **Speculum examination**
- Look for polyps, prolapsed fibroids, evidence of trauma, overt carcinoma.
- Look for bleeding point if secondary haemorrhage.
- Take swabs.

6 **Bimanual examination**
- Assess uterine size, tenderness, pelvic masses, cervical abnormalities.

7 **Arrange appropriate investigations**
- FBC, U&Es, coagulation studies, X-match four units (dependent on loss).
- Consider endometrial sampling/cervical biopsy if indicated.

8 **Consider need for urgent treatment to arrest bleeding**
- Vaginal packing (may need to be done in theatre).
- Suturing to local bleeding points.
- 'Emergency' curettage.

9 **Further management will depend on the suspected diagnosis**
- Is an ultrasound scan required?
- Will patient need elective hysteroscopy and endometrial sampling?
- Involve gynaecological oncologist or radiotherapist if underlying malignancy.

Severe dysfunctional uterine bleeding/menorrhagia

This occasionally presents as an acute emergency. It is commoner at the extremes of reproductive life (i.e. near the time of the menarche and also in the perimenopausal period). Medical treatment on an inpatient basis will usually be sufficient and subsequent treatment is entirely dependent on the patient's age etc. Occasionally, surgical intervention will be necessary to arrest haemorrhage.

1 **Resuscitate and transfuse as necessary**

2 **Institute medical treatment to arrest bleeding**
- High dose oral progesterone (e.g. norethisterone 10 mg tds or qds).
- Consider adding tranexamic acid 1 g qds po.
- Tranexamic acid 1 g tds may be administered by *slow intravenous infusion* in very severe cases.

3 **Consider need for urgent surgical intervention**
- Hysteroscopy and curettage.
- Balloon tamponade.

4 **Further investigations**
- Rarely, von Willebrand's disease or haematological malignancies such as acute myeloid leukaemia will present with severe menorrhagia.
- Does patient look hypothyroid?

5 **Consider treatment to maintain response**
- Tranexamic acid plus mefenamic acid (500 mg tds) during menstruation.
- Cyclical progesterone (e.g. norethisterone 5 mg tds days 5–25).
- GnRH analogues (e.g. goserelin 3.6 mg subcutaneously monthly).
- COCP.

6 **For cases of intractable haemorrhage**
- Consider arterial embolization.
- Rarely, emergency hysterectomy is required.

7 **Review need for further *elective* investigation**

SUPPLEMENTARY INFORMATION

Institute medical treatment to arrest bleeding

'Medical' curettage will be successful for most patients who should respond to high dose progesterone within 48 hours.

Consider need for urgent surgical intervention

If patient's condition worsens or bleeding does not settle, consider urgent surgical intervention. Surgical curettage may be necessary. Removal of a necrotic fibroid polyp may be required (see separate section below). Balloon tamponade may be considered, using a Foley catheter in a small cavity or a Sengstaken-Blakemore tube in a large cavity (balloon holds 300 ml). The Rusch urological hydrostatic catheter has a balloon capacity of 500 ml.

Intractable haemorrhage

Remember the uterus has an excellent collateral circulation but arterial embolization can reduce the haemorrhage to acceptable levels. Involve interventional radiologist.

Cervical polyp/fibroid polyp

Emergency admission can be the result of bleeding from a large, vascular endocervical polyp or a pedunculated fibroid polyp. In the latter case, there may be superimposed infection if the polyp is necrotic. Fibroid polyps can be very large, protruding through a dilated cervix which can be felt as a thin rim (on digital examination this feels similar to a dilated cervix applied to the fetal head in labour!).

MINI-ACTION PLAN FOR CERVICAL POLYP

1 **Vaginal packing may arrest acute haemorrhage**

2 **Consider removal on the ward only if the polyp has a thin pedicle**

3 **Remove polyp in theatre**
   - Grasp polyp with sponge forceps and avulse by twisting polyp on its pedicle. Diathermize the base.
   - Alternatively, remove using handheld diathermy needle or spade (useful if pedicle is thick or polyp is sessile on a broad base).

4 **If >40 years, consider hysteroscopy to exclude other polyps**

5 **Send any tissue removed for histological examination**

1 **Antibiotic cover if fibroid necrotic**

2 **Perform EUA and hysteroscopy (with equipment available for resection)**
- Define size and site of polyp base.
- Exclude other pathology.

3 **Remove fibroid polyp**
- If accessible, ligate the stalk of the fibroid as near to the base as possible with an 0 or 1 polyglactin suture before division with handheld diathermy.
- Handheld diathermy alone may be adequate (set on blend for cut/coagulation).
- If base is broad or inaccessible – use endometrial resection technique.

4 **Send fibroid for histology**

5 **Ensure haemostasis – use balloon tamponade if necessary (see above)**

Secondary haemorrhage after major surgery

Secondary haemorrhage with vaginal bleeding may follow major vaginal or abdominal pelvic surgery. It is always associated with underlying infection and can be heavy enough to lead to cardiovascular instability. Admission is usually on an emergency basis. If bleeding does not require immediate surgical intervention, manage conservatively.

1 **Resuscitate and transfuse as necessary**

2 **Take swabs (blood cultures as clinically indicated)**

3 **Commence broad spectrum antibiotics (iv if pyrexia >38°C, systemic sepsis or surgical intervention planned – e.g. cefuroxime 750 mg and metronidazole 500 mg, both iv 8 hourly or amoxycillin/potassium clavulanate 1.2 g iv 6–8 hourly)**

4 **Bleeding due to draining pelvic haematoma**
- Examine vaginally and define site of haematoma.
- Observation and conservative management.
- Majority of drainage usually subsides within 48 hours.

5 **Bleeding with fresh component**
- Consider vaginal packing with catheterization.
- Arrange examination in theatre if significant bleeding through pack.

6 **Examination under anaesthesia**
- Careful bimanual and speculum examination of vaginal walls and vault.
- Identify bleeding points and insert haemostatic sutures.
- Laparotomy is rarely required.

SUPPLEMENTARY INFORMATION

Examination under anaesthesia

Care should be taken in inserting deep haemostatic sutures near the vault angles to control bleeding as the ureters are at risk. Try and identify specific bleeding points, which will usually be in the vault edge. Laparotomy is often an unproductive exercise, revealing organizing haematoma in the pelvis with gross anatomical distortion. Specific bleeding points are rarely found. In extreme circumstances, large packs may be left in the pelvis and the abdomen closed. Repeat laparotomy is required 48 hours later for pack removal.

Bleeding due to malignancy

Heavy vaginal bleeding is usually related to cervical malignancy. Follow the previous action plan but consider involvement of gynaecological oncologist and interventional radiologist (arterial embolization). Endometrial carcinoma may first present with significant haemorrhage. High dose progesterone may control the bleeding but urgent hysteroscopy and surgical curettage may be required.

MINI ACTION PLAN – BLEEDING POST-LLETZ

1 **Resuscitate and transfuse as necessary**

2 **Take swabs (blood cultures as clinically indicated)**

3 **Commence broad spectrum antibiotics (iv if pyrexia >38.5°C, systemic sepsis or surgical intervention planned – e.g. cefuroxime 750 mg and metronidazole 500 mg, both iv 8 hourly or amoxicillin/ potassium clavulanate 1.2 g iv 6–8 hourly)**

4 **Conservative management if bleeding is not excessive**
- Observation only – expect bleeding to be settling within 12–24 hours.
- Vaginal packing with catheterization – remove pack in 12–24 hours.

5 **Surgical management if bleeding is excessive or not resolving**
- Consider assessment in colposcopy suite and diathermy (local anaesthetic).
- Consider assessment in theatre and haemostatic sutures (GA).

Non-Pregnant Causes of Vaginal Bleeding

MANAGEMENT OF THE EARLY PREGNANCY ASSESSMENT UNIT

Kim Hinshaw

The Early Pregnancy Assessment Unit or Clinic (EPAU or EPAC) allows efficient and effective management of women with early pregnancy bleeding or pain. Most women will avoid out of hours emergency admission with long periods away from friends and family. In the past, mean length of admission with bleeding in early pregnancy was 3 days. The average length of admission after EPAU assessment is only 1 day. Ideally, the service should run on a daily basis with individualized patient appointments. The appointments system should be accessible to all primary care health providers as well as other hospital departments (e.g. Accident & Emergency). The reduction in inpatient admissions can have significant economic benefits for the NHS.

PATIENTS SUITABLE FOR EPAU ASSESSMENT

- Vaginal bleeding in early pregnancy – light to moderate loss.
- Haemodynamically stable.
- If associated pain – should require no more than simple analgesics (e.g. paracetamol).
- Lower limit of gestation – 6+ weeks (with +ve urinary pregnancy test).
- Upper limit of gestation – usually 16–20 weeks.

Appointment should be available within 24 hours. EPAU is ideal for assessing those with a clinical diagnosis of threatened miscarriage, to confirm suspected complete miscarriage, to exclude suspected ectopic pregnancy (patient must be well with no severe localizing symptoms or signs), to offer reassurance to those with a previous history of ectopic or recurrent miscarriage.

STAFFING

Usually multidisciplinary and may involve all of the following:

- medical staff – SHO/SpR;
- nursing or midwifery staff (preferably with counselling skills);
- ultrasonographer.

ACTION PLAN

1 **Take history**
- Critically review the history of bleeding and relationship to any pain.
- Consider ectopic.
- Previous obstetric history.
- Was last menstrual period normal in onset and amount?
- When was pregnancy test performed?
- Cervical smear history.

2 **Take blood tests**

3 **General assessment and abdominal examination**

4 **Perform ultrasound scan – transabdominal (TA) +/– transvaginal (TV)**

5 **Consider need for speculum and bimanual pelvic examination**

6 **Allow time for discussion of diagnosis**
- Should occur in a suitable setting with support of partner (separate counselling room).
- If diagnosis is unclear at second EPAU visit, discuss case with senior staff.

7 **Arrange further management as appropriate**
- Viable – usually discharge to GP care.
- Indeterminate – arrange repeat ultrasound in 7–10 days.
- Miscarriage confirmed – discuss options (surgical, medical, expectant).
- Ectopic – usually offer laparoscopic surgery if stable. Some units use medical management (systemic methotrexate).

8 **Consider psychological care and need for follow-up**

CONSULT OTHER TOPICS

Complications of medical management for therapeutic abortion and miscarriage (p 96)
Complications of surgical management for therapeutic abortion and miscarriage (p 90)
Ectopic pregnancy (p 76)
Scan findings relevant to the Early Pregnancy Assessment Unit (p 68)

SUPPLEMENTARY INFORMATION

Take blood tests

Blood testing is often done near the start of the consultation in order to allow the laboratory time to check Rhesus status before the patient is discharged. Close liaison is needed between the EPAU and laboratory services. Serum hCG testing should be available on a daily basis to help in the diagnosis of asymptomatic ectopic pregnancy. The opportunity should be taken to check other routine pregnancy bloods (e.g. rubella, hepatitis, syphilis screen).

Perform ultrasound scan – TA +/– TV

Fifty to sixty percent of women attending the EPAU will need a TV scan in order to reach a diagnosis. Do not be tempted to leave out the TA scan. TV scan uses higher frequency (5–7.5 MHz) for improved definition, but has poorer penetration. Coexisting ovarian pathology may be missed with a TV scan if the ovaries are sited at the pelvic brim. TV scan is acceptable to patients in an early pregnancy setting.

Consider need for speculum and bimanual pelvic examination

Many women with a small threatened miscarriage do not need routine pelvic examination, particularly as they may be anxious at the time. However, women should be offered speculum/bimanual assessment in the following circumstances:

- heavy vaginal bleeding;
- suspected ectopic pregnancy (check for 'cervical excitation');
- significant pain;
- suspicion of 'products' in cervical canal;
- significant vaginal discharge;
- pelvic infection;
- recurrent episodes of bleeding (exclude rare causes: polyp, carcinoma).

Allow time for discussion of diagnosis

The following table outlines the likely diagnoses after a first visit to EPAU:

Diagnosis	Incidence
Threatened miscarriage (viable)	53%
Complete miscarriage	11%
Early fetal demise	4%
Incomplete miscarriage	3%
Indeterminate	22%
Suspected ectopic	3%
Not pregnant	4%

Consider psychological care and need for follow-up

Pregnancy loss can have a significant and long-lasting negative psychological impact for many women and their partners. All professionals should be aware of the need to offer continuing support. Follow-up should be offered in the EPAU or in primary care. The use of appropriate terminology is important (e.g. 'complete miscarriage' and not 'complete abortion').

FURTHER READING

Fox R, Richardson J and Sharma A (2000) Early pregnancy assessment. *Obst. Gynaecol.* **2(2):** 7–12.
Walker JJ and Shillito J (1997) Early pregnancy assessment units: service and organisational aspects. In: Grudzinskas JG and O'Brien PMS (eds), *Problems in Early Pregnancy: Advances in Diagnosis and Management.* RCOG Press, London, pp. 160–173.

SCAN FINDINGS RELEVANT TO THE EARLY PREGNANCY ASSESSMENT UNIT

Mamdouh Guirguis and Kim Hinshaw

An ultrasound scan is usually offered to all new patients attending the EPAU. Remember that over half of referred patients will have a viable pregnancy after assessment. The possibility of ectopic pregnancy should always be borne in mind in any patient with bleeding in early pregnancy. Up to 5% of referrals may turn out to be non-pregnant with other causes for their bleeding or abdominal pain. The recommended medical terminology which should be used in discussing miscarriage with patients will be used in this chapter.

TRANSABDOMINAL (TA) vs TRANSVAGINAL (TV) ULTRASOUND

TA probes use lower frequency (3.5 MHz) allowing better tissue penetration. TV probes use higher frequency (5–7.5 MHz) offering improved definition. Coexisting ovarian pathology and free fluid in the paracolic gutters may be missed with a TV scan. TV scanning can confirm viability at 4.5+ weeks (about 1 week earlier than TA scan). Overall, 50–60% of women attending the EPAU will need a transvaginal scan to reach a diagnosis. TA and TV scanning should be regarded as *complementary*.

STAFF UNDERTAKING ULTRASOUND ASSESSMENT

The sonographer may be a radiographer, nurse, midwife or doctor. They should be formally trained in both TA and TV ultrasound. Practice should follow the recommendations of the British Medical Ultrasound Society.

ACTION PLAN

The following action plan is common for all initial ultrasound assessments in the EPAU. It is followed by a series of mini-action plans relevant to each specific ultrasound diagnosis.

1 **Take history *before* ultrasound assessment**
   - Be aware of any symptoms which might suggest ectopic pregnancy (EP) – this may influence interpretation of scan findings.

2 **Speculum/pelvic examination is usually only required before scanning if there is *heavy bleeding***
   - Heavy bleeding (+/– pain) suggests inevitable or incomplete miscarriage and any tissue lodged in the cervical os can be removed prior to scanning.

3 **Perform TA ultrasound scan**

4 **Perform TV ultrasound scan if indicated**

5 **Review history, scan and pelvic findings**

6 Consider need for serum hCG assay to exclude ectopic

7 **Reach diagnosis – arrange further management as appropriate**
   - See mini action plans below.

CONSULT OTHER TOPICS

Complications of medical management for therapeutic abortion and miscarriage (p 96)
Complications of surgical management for therapeutic abortion and miscarriage (p 90)
Early pregnancy emergencies – admitting patients to the ward (p 73)
Ectopic pregnancy (p 76)
Management of the Early Pregnancy Assessment Unit (p 65)
Other causes of abdominal pain in early pregnancy (p 83)

SUPPLEMENTARY INFORMATION

Perform TA ultrasound scan

May give inconclusive results if empty bladder, maternal obesity, deep pelvis, uterine retroversion or early gestation. Review extrauterine findings, including pouch of Douglas and adnexal areas.

Reach diagnosis – arrange further management as appropriate

RCOG/RCR Working Party (1995) recommendations for scan reporting:

- 'viable intrauterine pregnancy';
- 'fetal pole; no cardiac activity';
- 'empty gestation sac';
- 'no gestation sac; probable retained products';
- 'empty uterus';
- 'suspected trophoblastic disease'.

The final clinical diagnosis will depend on the scan report plus other features from history and examination (+/– serum hCG).

Threatened miscarriage/viable intrauterine pregnancy

ACTION PLAN

1 **Scan report = 'viable intrauterine pregnancy'**

2 **Subchorionic haematoma – if sited under membranes = good prognosis**

3 **Embryonic heart rate – if *persistent* bradycardia = ↑ risk of miscarriage**

4 **Check need for anti-D immunoglobulin**

5 **Counsel – usually offered GP follow-up**

Inevitable miscarriage

ACTION PLAN

1 This is a clinical diagnosis – internal os open, but no tissue passed

2 Scan report = 'fetal pole; no cardiac activity' or 'empty gestation sac'. Occasionally 'viable intrauterine pregnancy' despite open os

3 **Additional scan features**
- Gestation sac positioned low in uterus.
- Dilated internal cervical os and canal.
- Bulging membranes through dilated cervix ('hour-glass').

4 **D/W patient – loss of pregnancy in first trimester is inevitable. Consider admission**

Non-viable intrauterine pregnancy – incomplete miscarriage

ACTION PLAN

1 If heavy bleeding, perform pelvic examination before scan

2 Scan report = 'No gestation sac; probable retained products'

3 **Additional scan features**
- Heterogenous shadows (mixed echogenicity) >15 mm maximum AP diameter.
- Cervical os may be open or closed.

4 **Arrange uterine evacuation (medical or surgical) unless bleeding minimal**

Non-viable intrauterine pregnancy – early fetal demise

ACTION PLAN

1 Scan report = 'fetal pole; no cardiac activity' or 'empty gestation sac'

2 **RCOG/RCR guidelines for definitive diagnosis of non-viability (TV scan)**
- CRL >6 mm with no fetal heart activity.
- Gestation sac empty with mean diameter >20 mm.

3 **Additional scan features**
- Sac outline irregular.
- Sac positioned low in uterus.
- Large sac relative to fetus.
- Large yolk sac (92% will miscarry if diameter >10 mm).

4 **D/W patient – offer uterine evacuation or conservative management**

5 **If patient unable to accept diagnosis – offer opportunity for repeat scanning**

Scan Findings Relevant to the EPAU

Non-viable intrauterine pregnancy – complete miscarriage

ACTION PLAN

1 **Scan report = 'empty uterus' (i.e. contains thin, well-defined midline echo)**

2 **Additional scan features**
- Uterus may contain heterogenous echoes <15 mm max AP diameter (vast majority will resolve with no intervention).

3 **Review clinical history – is ectopic likely? If YES – consider serial serum hCG +/– repeat scanning**

4 **D/W patient – if 'complete' miscarriage likely, offer conservative management (+/– repeat urine hCG in 7–10 days)**

Ectopic pregnancy (EP)

ACTION PLAN

1 **Scan report = 'empty uterus`**

2 **Additional scan features (PPV of the last three is ≤41%)**
- Adnexal ring with fetal pole (+/– FH activity).
- Free fluid in pouch of Douglas.
- 'Pseudo-sac` (may mimic intrauterine pregnancy).
- Adnexal mass.

3 **During scanning consider the following rarer sites of ectopic**
- Cornual.
- Heterotopic.
- Ovarian.
- Cervical.
- Abdominal.

4 **If definite tubal ectopic – arrange appropriate treatment (surgical or medical)**

5 **Review history and examination – is ectopic still a possibility? If YES – consider serial serum hCG +/– repeat scanning**

Gestational trophoblastic disease (GTD)

ACTION PLAN

1 **Scan report = 'suspected trophoblastic disease'**

2 **Additional scan features**
- Complete mole – uterus contains multiple cystic (sonolucent) spaces in a denser echogenic background (previously described as a 'snowstorm' appearance).
- Partial mole – may have a live fetus. Often triploid with severe early growth restriction. Some areas of placenta exhibit cystic change.
- Multiple theca lutein ovarian cysts (may be large).

3 **Check serum hCG. Institute appropriate management (usually surgical evacuation)**

Indeterminate ultrasound findings

1 **Scan diagnosis may be 'indeterminate' in 1/5 cases after first EPAU visit**
   - 'Fetal pole; no cardiac activity': if CRL <6 mm may be viable.
   - 'Empty gestation sac': if mean sac diameter <20 mm may be viable.
   - 'Empty uterus': some cases may reflect an EP.

2 **If indeterminate but potentially viable, repeat scan 7–10 days**

3 **Is ectopic likely? If YES – consider serial serum hCG (48 hour interval) +/– repeat scanning**

Scan Findings Relevant to the EPAU

EARLY PREGNANCY EMERGENCIES – ADMITTING PATIENTS TO THE WARD

Kim Hinshaw

The majority of patients referred with bleeding in early pregnancy, from primary care or Accident & Emergency, will be suitable for outpatient assessment in the EPAU or EPAC. However, a small proportion will still require urgent direct admission to the gynaecology ward for initial assessment or stabilization. After referral to the EPAU some patients will require direct ward admission, as will occasional cases from day theatre and other hospital departments (usually general surgical wards). Rarely, a patient may need to be transferred urgently to theatre from elsewhere in the hospital (e.g. haemodynamically unstable admissions to Accident & Emergency with incomplete miscarriage). This chapter reviews the groups of women who should still be urgently admitted to the gynaecology ward and their initial management.

PATIENTS UNSUITABLE FOR INITIAL EPAU ASSESSMENT (RECOMMEND WARD ADMISSION)

- Heavy vaginal bleeding in association with miscarriage.
- Significant pain in association with miscarriage.
- Unscheduled heavy bleeding during priming phase of medical evacuation for miscarriage.
- Suspected ectopic with significant abdominal pain.
- Suspected ectopic with signs of intraperitoneal bleeding (fainting, shoulder-tip pain or cervical excitation).
- Haemodynamic instability.
- Significant patient anxiety.
- Moderate pain/bleeding with poor social/home support or lack of transport.

ACTION PLAN

1 **If unstable – call for help and follow basic ABC of resuscitation**

2 **Initial rapid review of history and general assessment of condition**

3 **Take blood tests early whilst establishing venous access:**
- Full blood count (FBC).
- Group and save with antibody screen (check Rhesus status).
- X-match/clotting screen if clinically indicated.

4 **Abdominal examination**

5 **Speculum and bimanual pelvic examination as clinically indicated**

6 **Arrange further management as appropriate**
- Inform nursing staff of the plan of management.
- Plan further personal review as clinically indicated.
- Handover care to subsequent on-call emergency team.
- Ultrasound assessment can be arranged when clinically stable.

7 **Discuss case with senior staff (SpR or Consultant)**

CONSULT OTHER TOPICS

Cardiopulmonary resuscitation (p 234)
Complications of medical management for therapeutic abortion and miscarriage (p 96)
Complications of surgical management for therapeutic abortion and miscarriage (p 90)
Ectopic pregnancy (p 76)
Management of the Early Pregnancy Assessment Unit (p 65)

SUPPLEMENTARY INFORMATION

Initial rapid review of history and general assessment of condition

- Critical review of the history of bleeding or pain (ask relatives if present).
- Always consider ectopic.
- Previous pregnancy history.
- Was last menstrual period normal in onset, amount and duration?
- When was pregnancy test performed?

Speculum and bimanual pelvic examination as clinically indicated

It is still appropriate to admit a patient who is *extremely anxious*, even if bleeding is only light. These women may well decline pelvic examination at the time of admission. This can be deferred until after ultrasound assessment.

All other groups listed above should ideally have a pelvic assessment on admission. This will allow the admitting doctor to:

- assess the state of the cervical os (+/– removal of 'products' in cervical canal);
- take appropriate endocervical swabs for culture (including chlamydia);
- confirm uterine size;
- check for 'cervical excitation', tenderness or an obvious pelvic mass;
- exclude local causes for bleeding.

Patients undergoing uterine evacuation for miscarriage in daycase theatre – unplanned admission

Unscheduled admission from the dayunit theatre to the ward may be required in the following circumstances:

- significant haemorrhage (particularly if transfusion required);
- signs of significant pelvic infection or pyrexia;
- cervical trauma requiring suturing/packing;
- suspected perforation (laparoscopy or laparotomy undertaken);
- delayed recovery from anaesthesia;
- inability to void urine post-surgery;
- pain control inadequate to allow discharge;
- poor social/home support or lack of transport (nursing review only required).

1 Review by on-call team after transfer to ward

2 Check and record baseline observations, abdominal signs and vaginal bleeding

3 Initial discussion about reason for unscheduled admission with patient (+/– relatives). Record discussions

4 Inform nursing team of plan of management

5 Specify planned frequency of clinical observations

6 Plan further personal review as clinically indicated

7 Handover care to subsequent on-call team

ECTOPIC PREGNANCY

Mark Roberts, Niamh McCabe and Kim Hinshaw

The incidence of EP has increased markedly in the last few decades to 11.1 per 1000 pregnancies and it remains one of the major causes of maternal death. The Confidential Enquiries into Maternal Deaths in the UK (CEMD; 1997–1999) reports 12 deaths associated with EP, giving a death rate of 0.4 per 1000 EPs. There are well-established risk factors, the strongest risk being a history of previous EP, tubal surgery or *in-utero* diethystilboestrol exposure. EP rates are also strongly linked to trends in pelvic inflammatory disease and in particular Chlamydial infection. EP is associated with assisted reproductive techniques (e.g. IVF). **However, the diagnosis of EP should be considered in ALL women of reproductive age with abdominal pain, vaginal bleeding or collapse.**

Presentation varies from severe abdominal pain with shock to relatively asymptomatic women in the EPAC. The CEMD emphasizes a clear need to highlight common *atypical* clinical presentations, especially the way in which EP may mimic gastrointestinal disease. Diagnostic algorithms are now widely used and involve serum β-hCG estimation. Treatment options have been extended to include surgical, medical and conservative approaches.

CONSULT OTHER TOPICS

Acute abdominal pain (p 1)
Early pregnancy emergencies – admitting patients to the ward (p 73)
Management of the Early Pregnancy Assessment Unit (p 65)
Scan findings relevant to the Early Pregnancy Assessment Unit (p 68)
Upper tract pelvic infection (p 13)

Ruptured EP with collapse

Despite the advent of early pregnancy ultrasound and sensitive urinary pregnancy tests, women still occasionally present in a state of collapse from ruptured EP. This type of EP is often first seen by A&E staff.

ACTION PLAN

1 **Ensure plenty of help and institute ABCs of resuscitation**
   - Call gynaecology SpR. Inform senior staff.
   - Inform anaesthetist.

2 **Administer high-flow oxygen by mask**

3 **Insert two large-bore iv cannulae, and take blood for FBC, U&Es and X-match 6 units**

4 **Check urinary β-hCG – pass a catheter if necessary to obtain a specimen**
   - Modern tests are sensitive down to 25 miU/ml.
   - A correctly performed negative urinary pregnancy effectively rules out an EP.

5 **Infuse warmed crystalloid/colloid, but *do not waste time trying to normalize the blood pressure***

6 **Transfer urgently to theatre – do not waste time trying to get a scan**

7 **If evidence of haemodynamic compromise, proceed to immediate laparotomy**

8 **Make a Pfannenstiel incision and locate the bleeding tube manually (do not waste time packing etc.)**

9 **Applying a clamp across the ruptured tube will immediately stop the bleeding**

10 **Proceed to salpingectomy**
- Inspect the other tube – record appearance later.
- Wash out the abdomen with warmed saline.

11 **Review total blood loss with anaesthetist**
- Blood loss is usually *underestimated*.
- Consider insertion of central line in massive haemorrhage.
- Consider initial recovery in HDU/ITU if still unstable.

12 **Follow-up serum β-hCG is unnecessary for women who have undergone open salpingectomy**

13 **Do not forget to check Kleihauer and administer anti-D immunoglobulin in Rhesus-negative women**

SUPPLEMENTARY INFORMATION

In managing a woman with ruptured EP, the key point is to resuscitate at the same time as making urgent arrangements for theatre. These patients will often remain haemodynamically unstable until the abdomen is open and the bleeding tube clamped. In this situation do not defer moving to theatre in order to obtain a serum β-hCG or ultrasound scan. Occasionally, you may find that a bleeding corpus luteal cyst presents in exactly the same way and final diagnosis is made at laparotomy.

'Asymptomatic' EP – diagnosis

As EP is often suspected early in relatively asymptomatic women, all units must have diagnostic algorithms to aid diagnosis. The following action plan applies to those women who are being assessed in an EPAU, have undergone TV scan and fulfil the following criteria:

- relatively asymptomatic;
- urinary β-hCG positive;
- empty uterus or *small* 'indeterminate' intrauterine sac (?pseudo sac);
- 'ectopic pregnancy cannot be excluded with reasonable certainty'.

1 **Establish the last menstrual period (LMP) with as much certainty as possible**
   - Remember that 15% of women with EP describe no amenorrhoea.

2 **Perform pelvic examination**
   - Cervical excitation implies pelvic peritonism (blood or pus) and should not be ignored.
   - Exclude tenderness or a palpable mass.

3 **Take blood for β-hCG and group and antibody screen**

4 **If the β-hCG is >1500 IU/ml, and the uterus is empty, an EP is likely**
   - Increased likelihood if there is fluid in the pelvis, a complex adnexal mass, risk factors.
   - Treatment options are surgical, medical or conservative (see below).

5 **If the β-hCG is <1500 IU/ml with no significant clinical signs or symptoms – repeat in 48 hours**

6 **If the second β-hCG has doubled – arrange repeat TV scan**
   - An intrauterine pregnancy should be confirmed with serum β-hCG at this level.

7 **If the second β hCG has risen inadequately (i.e. has not approximately doubled) – EP is very likely**
   - Do not delay diagnosis because the patient is asymptomatic.
   - Discuss with senior staff to decide management (surgical, medical, conservative).

8 **If second β hCG has fallen, this suggests a 'failing pregnancy', but does not differentiate between intra- and extra-uterine gestations**
   - Rapid falls are associated with complete miscarriage.
   - Ensure follow-up to confirm urinary PT has become negative.
   - EPs can still rupture at low levels of serum β-hCG.

SUPPLEMENTARY INFORMATION

It is becoming increasingly common to diagnose EP before the onset of symptoms due to early referral and the development of early pregnancy assessment services. All gynaecology SpRs will be familiar with the scenario of the 'empty uterus' with a positive pregnancy test. Units should have management algorithms for this clinical situation. There is now a tendency for delayed diagnosis of EP in some patients who have multiple serum β-hCGs over a week or so, when the rise is inadequate. Remember – inadequate rise in serum β-hCG over *48 hours is the main diagnostic tool for EP in asymptomatic women.*

The majority of early EPs may resolve spontaneously. Options for treatment can include conservative, medical or surgical management. Which is chosen depends on various factors including symptoms, level of β-hCG, ultrasound findings, previous history, the woman's preferences and social situation, senior staff preference. Conservative or medical treatment does not require confirmation by diagnostic laparoscopy.

Surgical management of EP

Surgery remains the mainstay of management for EP. The wider use of laparoscopic surgery must be tempered by its use only in appropriate circumstances by appropriately trained surgeons (CEMD 1997–1999).

1 **Establish iv access, FBC, G&S**

2 **Discuss surgical options with patient**
- Laparoscopic approach is recommended for most patients – always confirm that open surgery may be required.
- Laparoscopic salpingectomy is the treatment of choice if the contralateral tube is normal.
- Laparoscopic linear salpingotomy should be attempted if the contralateral tube is absent or abnormal.

3 **Linear salpingotomy – technique**
- Incise over ectopic with needle diathermy.
- Evacuate EP – hydrodissection may lead to less bleeding than removing EP 'piecemeal'.
- Diathermize bleeding points.
- Salpingotomy incision in Fallopian tube does not require suturing.

4 **Linear salpingotomy – follow-up**
- Persistent trophoblast occurs in 15% of women after laparoscopic salpingotomy.
- Repeat urine pregnancy test 1 week post-surgery and arrange serum β-hCG if positive.
- Persistent trophoblast is usually managed by repeat surgery or methotrexate (MTX).

5 **Complete comprehensive operative note in all cases**
- Particularly note the state of remaining Fallopian tube etc.
- Record blood loss.
- Outline plan for post-operative management and follow-up.

6 **Do not forget to check Kleihauer and administer anti-D immunoglobulin in Rhesus-negative women**

SUPPLEMENTARY INFORMATION

Discuss surgical options with patient

If mild adhesions are noted around the contralateral tube, they may be divided. It is not appropriate to embark on prolonged tubal surgery in the acute situation. Certain patients may request 'sterilization' of the contralateral tube at the time of emergency surgery. In most cases, this is probably not appropriate as the implications of permanent sterilization require careful consideration. However, management should be individualized (i.e. the process may be considered with an unexpected ectopic in a woman >40 years using an IUCD). All cases should be discussed with senior staff before proceeding. For women with a previous sterilization who present with EP – salpingectomy with repeat clipping of the contralateral tube is usual. Bilateral salpingectomy may be considered.

Medical management of EP

Medical treatment with methotrexate is an alternative option in selected women. It is particularly appropriate for women with significant surgical risk such as obesity and previous surgery. It is not indicated for women with significant symptoms or haemodynamic changes who need urgent surgical intervention. It is not suitable for women with high levels of β-hCG (>10 000 IU/ml) or large ectopic pregnancies (>3.5 cm) as the failure rate of medical treatment is higher in these women. Medical treatment should not be used where co-operation with follow-up is in doubt.

ACTION PLAN

1 **Discuss management plan**
   - Include potential side-effects (rare but serious – 'Stevens-Johnson').
   - Need for follow-up for 2–3 weeks to monitor fall in β-hCG.

2 **Take blood for β-hCG, FBC, group & antibodies, U&Es and LFTs**
   - Methotrexate is contraindicated in women with renal or hepatic impairment.

3 **Admit and obtain iv access – plan overnight stay**

4 **Administer 50 mg/m² of methotrexate im**
   - Consider safety aspects – ?administer on chemotherapy day unit.

5 **Prescribe simple analgesia**
   - Moderate increase in pain is common in the first 24 hours.
   - Any pain not controlled by simple analgesics or associated with haemodynamic compromise suggests tubal rupture and requires urgent surgical intervention.

6 **Monitor β-hCG on days 4, 7, 10 and then weekly until β-hCG is <15 IU/ml**
   - An initial increase is to be expected between day 1 and day 4.
   - This can also be associated with an increase in pain.
   - Expect a decrease in serum β-hCG of 15% between tests.
   - If <15% repeat the same dose of methotrexate (15% will require a second injection).

7 **Allow 'open access' to the gynaecology ward**
   - Rarely, tubal rupture can occur despite falling β-hCG levels.

8 **Do not forget to check Kleihauer and administer anti-D immunoglobulin in Rhesus-negative women**

Conservative management of EP

Up to 30% of women with an EP have declining β-hCG levels at presentation, and up to 85% of those with an initial β-hCG <200 IU/ml will resolve spontaneously. Patient should be relatively asymptomatic with no signs of intraperitoneal bleeding on ultrasound scan.

1 **Discuss diagnosis and management plan with patient**
- With spontaneously resolving trophoblast it may be impossible to be certain of the site of the pregnancy.
- Advise re-admission if symptoms develop or worsen.

2 **Check serum β-hCG weekly until < 50 IU/ml**
- Confirm negative urine PT thereafter.

3 **Allow 'open access' to the gynaecology ward**

4 **Consider medical or surgical management if rate of decline of β-hCG is slow or symptoms develop**

5 **Do not forget to check Kleihauer and administer anti-D immunoglobulin in Rhesus-negative women**

Non-tubal EP

Most EPs are tubal, and those which occur elsewhere pose difficult management problems.

Cervical EP

This may present with massive vaginal bleeding, or be detected on ultrasound.

1 **If collapsed follow ABCs and resuscitate as for ruptured tubal EP**

2 **Consider tamponade with a 'Rusch' urological balloon for life-threatening haemorrhage (insert and inflate in cervical canal)**

3 **Consider conservative options**
- Discuss arterial embolization with interventional radiologist before embarking on curettage.
- Surgery – curettage (may be associated with significant haemorrhage requiring Rusch ballon at end of procedure – alternatively conventional packing).

4 **Abdominal hysterectomy**
- For intractable haemorrhage after conservative approach.
- May be considered as primary treatment if future fertility is not an issue.

5 **Cervical pregnancy may be managed medically, but must be as an in-patient**

Cornual EP

1 **Rare and often diagnosed late**
- Consider diagnosis when pain is greater than expected.
- May present with rupture in mid-trimester.

2 **If collapsed follow ABCs and resuscitate as for ruptured tubal EP**

3 **Laparotomy, salpingectomy and cornual resection**
- Resect cornua with a wedge incision.
- Vascular procedure.
- Use deep 'figure of eight' haemostatic sutures to close (No '1' polyglactin).

4 **Very high level of skill required to perform cornual resection laparo-scopically**

5 **MTX for women diagnosed early on ultrasound, who are haemody-namically stable**

Heterotopic pregnancy

Previously very rare. However, the co-existence of intra- and extrauterine pregnancies occurs in up to 1% of assisted reproduction conceptions. Consider the diagnosis in these circumstances.

ACTION PLAN

1 **Laparoscopic salpingectomy is the treatment of choice**
- Survival of the intrauterine pregnancy is better with surgical management.

2 **Systemic methotrexate is contraindicated**
- If strong indications for medical treatment, 1 ml of 20% potassium chloride may be injected into the ectopic gestation sac.

3 **Follow-up with serial ultrasound**
- β-hCG is not possible because of the ongoing pregnancy.

4 **Do not forget to check Kleihauer and administer anti-D immunoglobulin in Rhesus-negative women**

Ovarian EP

ACTION PLAN

1 **Rare and diagnosis may be delayed**
- Consider diagnosis when pain continues after negative laparoscopy.
- May present with massive intraperitoneal haemorrhage.

2 **If collapsed follow ABCs and resuscitate as for ruptured tubal EP**

3 **Surgical treatment with unilateral salpingo-oophorectomy**
- Laparoscopic or open approach may be required.

4 **Diagnosis is confirmed histologically**

REFERENCES

Ankum WM, Mol BW, Van der Veen F *et al.* (1996) Risk factors for ectopic pregnancy: a meta-analysis. *Fertil. Steril.* **65**: 1093–1099.
Clinical greentop guidelines – the management of tubal pregnancies. RCOG, London. www.rcog.org.uk/guidelines.asp?PageID=106&GuidelineID=22
Lipscomb GH, Stovall TH and Ling FW (2000) Nonsurgical treatment of ectopic pregnancy. *NEJM* **243(18)**: 1325–1329.

OTHER CAUSES OF ABDOMINAL PAIN IN EARLY PREGNANCY

Kim Hinshaw

Abdominal pain in early pregnancy is common and has many causes which may or may not be pregnancy-related. It is a cause of significant anxiety for pregnant women who will often feel that any abdominal pain is a potential sign of miscarriage. However, in many cases the cause is not serious. For those women admitted on an emergency basis, the following action plan and discussion should help the clinician to reach a prompt diagnosis and allow appropriate reassurance to be given at the earliest opportunity. As with all emergency cases, the importance of a thorough history and examination, cannot be over-emphasized.

ACTION PLAN

1 **Take accurate history**
- Critically review the history of pain – onset, nature, duration, radiation etc.
- Consider EP.
- Relationship of pain to any bleeding.
- Previous obstetric history.
- Previous surgical and medical history.

2 **General and abdominal examination**

3 **Pelvic examination**

4 **Arrange appropriate investigations**

5 **Differential diagnosis – consider pregnancy-related or gynaecological causes**

Pregnancy related	Gynaecological causes
Common	
Tubal EP	Ovarian cyst accident
Miscarriage	Acute urinary retention
Hyperemesis gravidarum	
Rare	
Cornual or ovarian ectopic	Pelvic infection
Ruptured rudimentary horn	Fibroid torsion or degeneration
Septic abortion	Torsion of fimbrial cyst

Surgical	Medical
Common	
Appendicitis	Urinary tract infection
Ureteric calculus	Constipation
Gastric reflux	Irritable bowel syndrome
Rare	
Peptic ulceration	Threadworm infestation
Cholecystitis	Diverticulitis
Pancreatitis	Sickle cell crisis
Inflammatory bowel disease	Porphyria
Obstruction / volvulus	
Meckel's diverticulitis	
Subrectus haematoma	

7 **Further management**
- When the diagnosis remains unclear – regular and critical review should be undertaken.
- This should involve surgical colleagues as dictated by clinical suspicion.

CONSULT OTHER TOPICS

Acute abdominal pain (p 1)
Early pregnancy emergencies – admitting patients to the ward (p 73)
Ectopic pregnancy (p 76)
Scan findings relevant to the Early Pregnancy Assessment Unit (p 65)
Surgical management of ovarian cysts in the pregnant and non-pregnant (p 6)

SUPPLEMENTARY INFORMATION

General and abdominal examination

The woman with abdominal pain in early pregnancy will often be admitted under the care of the gynaecologist, who should always be particularly aware of the surgical or medical conditions that should be considered.

Review the patient's general condition and note any pyrexia. A critical history of the pain should be taken. Consider the different types of abdominal pain.

Visceral pain

This is felt centrally and is often dull and poorly localized. Midgut pain (duodenojejunal junction to midtransverse colon) is usually peri-umbilical and hindgut pain (midtransverse colon to anorectal junction) is felt in the central lower abdomen. This can be difficult to differentiate from uterine or bladder-related pain.

Peritoneal pain

This is somatic and well-localized to the site of the organ of origin. It tends to be more severe.

Pelvic examination

During assessment of the cervix, uterus and adnexal areas to exclude EP, careful consideration should be given to other causes of unilateral pelvic mass (ovarian cyst, fimbrial cyst) and cervical excitation. This latter sign may be found whenever there is pelvic peritoneal irritation by blood or pus. Ovarian cyst rupture and appendicitis should be considered (acute pelvic infection is extremely unusual in pregnancy).

Arrange appropriate investigations

Will depend on differential diagnosis, but usually requires:

- FBC – note WCC >15 x 10^9/l;
- urea and electrolytes;
- MSU – microscopy, culture and sensitivity;
- ultrasound of pelvis – uterine contents, adnexal masses, free fluid (pelvis or paracolic gutters);
- serum amylase/LFTs – if pain is peri-umbilical or upper abdominal.

Differential diagnosis – consider pregnancy-related or gynaecological causes

The causes which are not described in other chapters are reviewed below:

- *Acute urinary retention* often in association with a retroverted uterus in late first trimester. Short term catheterization required. If recurs will usually resolve by 14 weeks.
- *Hyperemesis gravidarum* – severe vomiting may lead to pain from upper GIT or musculoskeletal from abdominal wall.
- *Fibroid torsion or degeneration* – fibroids occur in 0.5–1.0% of pregnancies and increase in size in early pregnancy. Risk of torsion if pedunculated. 'Red' degeneration and localized pain occurs if blood supply is outgrown. Manage conservatively with analgesics.
- *Torsion of fimbrial cyst* – rare. Presents like a torted ovarian cyst.
- *Ruptured rudimentary horn* – rare. Continuing severe uterine pain. Likely to rupture midtrimester.

Differential diagnosis – consider other causes: surgical and medical

- *Appendicitis* – most common general surgical emergency in pregnancy (1 in 2000). Diagnosis is more difficult as pregnancy progresses – site of maximal tenderness moves upwards and laterally in midtrimester. Important to operate before perforation as this increases risk of miscarriage.
- *Ureteric calculus/urinary tract infection* – History of previous UTI or calculi should be sought. Commonly lower tract infection in early pregnancy. Upper tract UTI is more commonly right-sided. Passage of calculi invariably associated with detectable haematuria. Most stones will pass spontaneously. Use opioid analgesia as indicated.
- *Gastric reflux/peptic ulceration (PU)* – the former is common and the latter rare. Previous history of PU prior to pregnancy. PU may be difficult to diagnose as upper GI symptoms are common in pregnancy.
- *Constipation/irritable bowel syndrome* – bowel colic usually improves with the raised progesterone levels of pregnancy. Acute episodes may occur as women may avoid their usual antispasmodic medication.

Other Causes of Abdominal Pain in Early Pregnancy

- *Cholecystitis* – usually past history of attacks. Laparoscopic approach suitable if intervention required in early pregnancy.
- *Pancreatitis* – consider as differential with severe, acute onset upper abdominal pain. Amylase levels as per non-pregnant.
- *Inflammatory bowel disease* – if diagnosed, usually improves with pregnancy. May present with blood/mucus rectally, altered bowel habit and colicky pain. Common in fertile age group – Crohn's commoner in females. 10% have a first degree relative affected.
- *Obstruction/volvulus.* Volvulus accounts for 25% of obstruction occurring in pregnancy. Herniae should be considered – appropriate sites examined. Umbilical herniae can appear in pregnancy.
- *Meckel's diverticulitis* – "2% population, 2 inches long, 2 feet from ileocaecal junction". May mimic acute appendicitis.
- *Subrectus haematoma* – can occur spontaneously. Severe, localized superficial pain. Mass is not always evident.
- *Threadworm infestation* – commoner when there are other young children in the home. Often pain is more chronic and colicky. Can be a cause of acute appendicitis.
- *Sickle cell crisis* – usually diagnosed pre-pregnancy. Homozygous state may result in severe crisis precipitated by infection.
- *Porphyria* – although rare, may present for the first time during pregnancy. Be aware of association with hypertension, disorientation, dark urine. Manage conservatively with aggressive rehydration and analgesia.
- *Diverticulitis* – rare in this age group.

Further management

When common pregnancy-related and gynaecological conditions have been excluded, management should involve other specialties at an early stage. If a surgical diagnosis is considered, regular and repeated review by both teams should be undertaken as it can frequently take longer to reach a final diagnosis in pregnancy.

FURTHER READING

Knudsen UB and Aagaard J (1998) Acute plevic pain. In: Studd J (ed) *Progress in Obstetrics and Gynaecology*, Volume 13. Churchill Livingstone, London, pp. 311–323.

Mortensen NJ McC (2000) The small and large intestines. In: Russell RCG, Williams NS and Bulstrode CJK (eds) *Bailey & Love`s Short Practice of Surgery*. Arnold, London, pp. 1026–1057.

O`Herlihy C (1999). The acute abdomen in pregnancy. In: Monson J, Duthie G and O`Malley K (eds) *Surgical Emergencies*. Blackwell Science, Oxford, pp. 384–391.

THERAPEUTIC ABORTION – INDICATIONS AND THE ABORTION ACT

Kim Hinshaw

The Abortion Act 1967, came into effect on 27 April 1968. Various amendments have been made, the last (No 499) in 1991. 183 250 abortion procedures were undertaken in England and Wales in 1999. The trend in the abortion rate continues to rise (13–14 per 1000 women aged 15–44). The Maternal Mortality Report for 1994–1996 described one death related to therapeutic abortion. Death rates are detailed below. Importantly, there have been no reported deaths from *illegal abortion* in the last five triennial reports.

Direct deaths related to therapeutic abortion, UK 1985–1996

Triennium	Legal abortion	Illegal abortion	Approx rate/ 10^6 maternities
1985–1987	1	0	0.5
1988–1990	3	0	1.3
1991–1993	5	0	2.2
1994–1996	1	0	0.5

The following action plan includes the administrative steps which must be completed, before starting a therapeutic abortion. Note the exceptions described for 'emergency' abortion.

1 **Take history**
- Confirm LMP.
- Review contraceptive use (include plans for future contraception).
- Review social situation, family and peer support.
- Have all three options been considered (i.e. abortion, keep baby, adoption)?
- Confirm patient requests termination of her own volition.
- Confirm patient is sure of her decision.
- Record reasons for choosing termination.

2 **Examination**

3 **Arrange appropriate investigations**

4 **Relevant documentation completed**

5 **Obtain informed consent**
- Verbal discussion of procedure and risks (use information leaflets to support).
- Confirm patient is ready to make decision.
- Obtain written consent.

6 **Communicate with co-professionals**

CONSULT OTHER TOPICS

Consent (p 279)

Complications of medical management for therapeutic abortion and miscarriage (p 96)

Complications of surgical management for therapeutic abortion and miscarriage (p 90)

Risk management for medical staff (p 276)

Termination of pregnancy and maternal cardiac disease (p 101)

SUPPLEMENTARY INFORMATION

Examination

Offer speculum examination to screen for STDs (see next section). If ultrasound not available, undertake bimanual pelvic examination to estimate uterine size and position: *retroversion* is associated with an increased risk of uterine perforation at the time of surgical abortion.

Arrange appropriate investigations

Blood tests

FBC, blood group (including Rhesus) and antibody testing are mandatory. Consider other pregnancy screening blood tests as per local guidelines (rubella, syphilis, hepatitis, HIV).

Chlamydial screening

Recommended for all patients undergoing termination (specific test as per local policy). Consider screening with endocervical swabs for other infections (including gonorrhoea).

Opportunistic cervical cytology screening

Consider if >20 years and no screening in previous 3–5 years (dependent on local screening interval).

Ultrasound assessment

Not mandatory for management of termination but can provide the following information:

- accurate estimate of gestation;
- diagnosis of non-viable pregnancy;
- diagnosis of multiple pregnancy;
- uterus empty – consider ?not pregnant ?ectopic;
- incidental ovarian pathology.

Ultrasound assessment was recommended in the last Maternal Mortality Report. Accurate estimation of gestation may affect the type of termination offered. Confirmation of an unsuspected non-viable pregnancy removes the need to request a formal termination.

Relevant documentation completed

The Abortion Act requires Form HSA1 (Certificate A) to be completed before a termination is performed. The certificate is now produced on white paper (previously printed on blue). In normal circumstances, this must be done by two independent, registered medical practitioners. The patient's request must fulfil one or more of the specific circumstances below:

A. the continuance of the pregnancy would involve risk to the life of the pregnant woman greater than if the pregnancy were terminated;
B. the termination is necessary to prevent grave permanent injury to the physical or mental health of the pregnant woman;
C. the pregnancy has NOT exceeded its 24th week and that the continuance of the pregnancy would involve risk, greater than if the pregnancy were terminated, of injury to the physical or mental health of the pregnant women;
D. the pregnancy has NOT exceeded its 24th week and that the continuance of the pregnancy would involve risk, greater than if the pregnancy were terminated, of injury to the physical or mental health of any existing child(ren) of the family of the pregnant woman;
E. there is substantial risk that if the child were born it would suffer from such physical or mental abnormalities as to be seriously handicapped.

The operating practitioner **may certify alone** in the following emergency circumstances:

F. to save the life of the pregnant woman;
G. to prevent grave permanent injury to the physical or mental health of the pregnant woman.

Amendment 449 (1991) introduced a time limit of 24 weeks under grounds C and D, whilst A, B and E are *without time limit*.

Obtain informed consent

If under 16 years, a patient may give consent under the Gillick principle if deemed competent to understand the full implications of the procedure (including risks). In these circumstances, the operator can proceed without parental consent but must first emphasize and record the importance of parental support to the young woman.

Communicate with co-professionals

Include appropriate support services (e.g. social worker, counsellor) as well as patient's GP (assuming patient gives consent).

FURTHER READING

Abortion statistics (2000) Legal abortions carried out under the 1967 Abortion Act in England & Wales, 1999. ONS, London.
Why Mothers Die (1998) Report on confidential enquiries into maternal deaths in the United Kingdom 1994–1996. HMSO, London.

COMPLICATIONS OF SURGICAL MANAGEMENT FOR THERAPEUTIC ABORTION AND MISCARRIAGE

Kim Hinshaw

Surgical techniques are used in 88% of abortions undertaken on UK residents. Of these, 92% are managed by vacuum aspiration termination (VAT) and the rest at later gestations, by Dilatation and Evacuation (D&E) +/– VAT. In 2000, very few women were managed by hysterotomy or hysterectomy (*n* = 26). Surgical uterine evacuation remains the mainstay of management for incomplete and missed miscarriage and usually involves a vacuum aspiration method (also known as 'suction evacuation'). In this chapter, action plans are discussed for the management of significant complications associated with surgically emptying the uterus.

CONSULT OTHER TOPICS

Complications of medical management for therapeutic abortion and miscarriage (p 96)
Septic shock (p 267)
Termination of pregnancy and maternal cardiac disease (p 101)
Therapeutic abortion – indications and the Abortion Act (p 87)
Upper tract pelvic infection (p 13)

VAT/SUCTION EVACUATION OF THE UTERUS

The techniques used for evacuation of the uterus for miscarriage and therapeutic abortion are essentially the same. Previously, incomplete miscarriage was managed by curettage with a blunt or sharp metal curette. However, RCT evidence suggests that suction methods are easier and safer for incomplete miscarriage. The main complications to consider are: cervical trauma, uterine perforation, primary haemorrhage, secondary haemorrhage/infection and septic abortion. These will be reviewed in the following action plans.

CERVICAL TRAUMA

ACTION PLAN

Trauma may involve tearing of the cervix by applied instruments or damage to the internal cervical os by excessive or inappropriate dilatation. The latter may increase future obstetric risk (midtrimester loss and preterm delivery).

1 **Reduce risks of cervical trauma – pre-operative**
- Consider ultrasound assessment of gestation.
- Appropriate cervical preparation.
- Prostaglandin (PG) analogues are more effective than osmotic dilators.

2 **Reduce risks of cervical trauma – intra-operative**
- Grasp cervix with TWO vulsellum tenacula.

- Use graduated dilators.
- Dilate against appropriate counter-traction.

3 Management of cervical tears
- If small and not bleeding – no action.
- If large or bleeding – haemostatic polyglactin suture(s).
- May require packing and admission for overnight observation.

SUPPLEMENTARY INFORMATION

Reduce risks of cervical trauma – pre-operative

Young, nulliparous patients are at particular risk. RCT evidence has confirmed that PG analogues are more effective than osmotic dilators and significantly reduce the pressure required to dilate the cervix. This may protect the internal cervical os. Appropriate regimens are: 600–800 µg misprostol or 1 mg gemeprost inserted into posterior fornix 3 hours pre-operatively.

Reduce risks of cervical trauma – intra-operative

Using two vulsellum tenacula, distributes traction over a wider area. The teeth are blunt or grooved, reducing the risk of tissue puncture compared to use of a single-toothed tenaculum. The commonly used 'Hegar' dilators are round-ended but are not graduated – they require greater dilatation force. 'Hawkins-Amblers' dilators are one type of graduated dilator. Dilatation should be kept to a minimum. A good working rule is to achieve dilatation in millimetres equivalent to (or 1 mm more than) the gestation in weeks. Prior ultrasound assessment may thus prevent excessive dilatation when clinical examination overestimates gestation.

UTERINE PERFORATION

ACTION PLAN

The incidence of perforation is approximately 0.5% but associated bowel trauma is less common (0.15%).

1 Reduce risks of perforation – pre-operative
- Pelvic examination in clinic – diagnose retroversion.
- Ultrasound assessment of gestation (can also delineate ante- or retroversion).
- Consider cervical preparation with PG analogues.

2 Reduce risks of perforation – intra-operative
- Examine under anaesthesia *before* instrumentation.
- Catheterize if bladder impedes adequate examination.
- Use counter-traction to straighten cervical canal and reduce ante/retroversion.
- Use graduated dilators.
- DO NOT sound the uterus.
- Minimize number of instruments inserted into uterus.
- Insert suction cannula with the sliding sleeve OPEN.
- Be aware that the uterus will contract and cavity shorten during procedure.

3 **When to suspect perforation**
- In association with 'difficult' dilatation.
- Signs may be minimal – slight loss of resistance having reached the fundus, instruments passing further than expected.
- No tissue obtained with curette inserted appropriate distance.
- 'Unusual' bits of tissue seen (?bowel mucosa, appendix epiploica, omentum).
- *Perforation has occurred* when a bowel loop or omentum is brought down.

4 **Management of perforation/suspected perforation**

a **Inform anaesthetist of your suspicions (will insert large bore iv cannula)**

b **CALL EARLY for senior help**

c **DO NOT repeatedly insert instruments to check:**
- in particular, avoid repeated application of suction.

d **If in doubt – perform laparoscopy**

e **If 'simple' uterine perforation at laparoscopy (fundal perforation, minimal bleeding, no obvious bowel trauma):**
- end procedure and observe for 24 hours minimum;
- consider antibiotic prophylaxis.

f **After discharge – REMEMBER that bowel perforation may present late (i.e. after several days):**
- offer patient appropriate advice and open access to ward.

g **If haemorrhage is not settling at laparoscopy:**
- repair perforation;
- laparoscopically or via laparotomy (depends on skill of operator).

h **If 'suspicious' of bowel damage at laparoscopy:**
- proceed to laparotomy (use vertical incision);
- contact general surgeon;
- give antibiotic prophylaxis (iv cefuroxime and metronidazole).

SUPPLEMENTARY INFORMATION

Reduce risks of perforation – pre-operative

If ultrasound is not available, undertake bimanual pelvic examination to estimate uterine size and position: *retroversion and retroflexion* are associated with an increased risk of uterine perforation. Ultrasound is not mandatory for management of termination but can provide the following useful information:

- accurate estimate of gestation;
- unsuspected retroversion;
- unsuspected non-viable pregnancy;
- multiple pregnancy;
- empty uterus – consider ectopic (or not pregnant!);
- incidental ovarian pathology.

Reduce risks of perforation – intra-operative

Bimanual examination is essential to exclude retroversion. The uterine sound is the smallest diameter instrument on the standard tray and is associated with 23% of perforations. The suction curette is designed to empty the uterus. Although some operators perform a final 'security check' with a metal curette to confirm that the cavity is 'empty', this is responsible for up to 31% of perforations. Therefore, routine uterine sounding and use of a metal curette are not recommended.

PRIMARY HAEMORRHAGE

The incidence of reported haemorrhage for therapeutic abortion is 1.34 per 1000 procedures but may be higher due to under-reporting.

1 **Reduce risk of haemorrhage – pre-operative**
- Use of PG analogues significantly reduces amount of bleeding.

2 **Reduce risks of haemorrhage – intra-operative**
- Appropriate use of suction curette.
- 'Rub-up' compression bimanually.
- Consider oxytocics.

3 **Intractable haemorrhage**
- Call for help/inform senior staff.
- Anaesthetist to arrange urgent X-match.
- Oxytocics.
- Consider possibility of perforation.
- Consider packing uterus or 'Foley' catheter/'Rusch' balloon tamponade.
- Rarely – laparotomy and hysterectomy.

SUPPLEMENTARY INFORMATION

Reduce risks of haemorrhage – intraoperative

Rotatory movement of the curette creates a vortex which will remove bulky tissue (placenta). In-and-out movements produce strong pulling effects for removing lodged tissue. Ensure tubing is not blocked and recheck cavity if bleeding continues. The following drugs may be required. Intravenous ergometrine 500 µg stat or iv syntocinon bolus 10 IU (latter may cause hypotension). Intravenous syntocinon infusion (40 units in 500 ml 0.9% saline at 125 ml/h).

SECONDARY HAEMORRHAGE/INFECTION

This usually reflects underlying infection rather than retained tissue. Most cases will respond to appropriate broad spectrum antibiotics. RCT evidence confirms a significant reduction in post-termination pelvic infection with routine screening for chlamydia and antibiotic prophylaxis for all women (swab +ve or –ve).

1 **Speculum and bimanual pelvic examination (including endocervical swabs)**

2 **FBC (WCC), group & save, iv access as appropriate**

3 **Start broad spectrum antibiotics**
- Oral or iv dependent on clinical condition.
- If condition allows, review after 12–24 hours of antibiotic therapy.
- Discharge home if bleeding settling, otherwise arrange ultrasound scan.

4 **Pelvic ultrasound scan**
- Heterogenous shadows may imply retained products, decidua or blood clot.
- Surgical evacuation if AP diameter >15 mm or if significant bleeding continues.

5 **MINI-ACTION PLAN – Severe haemorrhage**
a Institute ABCs of resuscitation
b Call for help / inform senior staff
c Oxytocics
d IV broad spectrum antibiotics
e Arrange urgent surgical curettage (must be an experienced operator)
f If bleeding continues despite curettage – consider packing uterus or 'Foley' catheter / 'Rusch' balloon tamponade / uterine artery embolization
g Rarely – laparotomy and hysterectomy

SEPTIC ABORTION

Although uncommon in the UK, the possibility of illegal abortion should be considered. May present with septic shock and associated multi-organ failure and high mortality. Review the chapter discussing management of septic shock (p 267). Multidisciplinary approach involving intensivist, microbiologist and anaesthetist. Surgical evacuation may be considered after 24 hours of antibiotics and must be undertaken by senior staff. See previous section for management of severe haemorrhage.

Midtrimester surgical techniques (including hysterotomy and hysterectomy)

For the majority of practicing gynaecologists in the UK, medical techniques using combinations of antiprogesterone and PG analogues offer the most appropriate approach for management of midtrimester abortion or miscarriage. Midtrimester surgical techniques require greater surgical skill. The reported complications associated with termination increase with gestation: <13 weeks = 2.1 per 1000; 13–19 weeks = 4.6 per 1000; 20+ weeks = 9.8 per 1000. The majority of these are related to haemorrhage and uterine perforation. This action plan reviews a safe approach to midtrimester surgical uterine evacuation. This technique should not be undertaken without adequate training.

1 **Prior screening for chlamydial infection**

2 **Confirm gestation by ultrasound scan**

3 **Prepare cervix prior to surgery**
- PG analogues (see above).
- Osmotic dilators.

4 **Careful cervical dilatation**

5 **Evacuation under ultrasound control**

6 **Use appropriate instruments**

7 **Ensure haemostasis**
- Risk of haemorrhage increases with increasing gestation.
- Additional oxytocics may be necessary.

8 **Confirm major fetal parts are completely removed**
- This is the responsibility of the operating surgeon.
- Should be undertaken before anaesthetic is reversed.

9 **Don't forget to check Kleihauer and administer anti-D immunoglobulin in Rhesus-negative women**

SUPPLEMENTARY INFORMATION

Evacuation under ultrasound control

Routine use of ultrasound has been shown to reduce the incidence of uterine perforation.

Use appropriate instruments

This includes sponge-holding (ring) forceps for removing substantial fetal parts. Fetus will be dismembered. Cavity may be checked at end of procedure with large (12 mm) vacuum curette.

REFERENCES

Abortion Statistics Annual Reference volume – Series AB 27 (2001) Legal abortions carried out under the 1967 Abortion Act in England & Wales, 2000. ONS, London. www.statistics.gov.uk

Hinshaw K and Fayyad A (2000) *The management of early pregnancy loss*. RCOG 'Greentop' guideline No 25. RCOG, London.

Induced abortion (1997). RCOG 'Greentop' guideline No 11. RCOG, London.

COMPLICATIONS OF MEDICAL MANAGEMENT FOR THERAPEUTIC ABORTION AND MISCARRIAGE

Kim Hinshaw

Early medical therapeutic abortion has been available in the UK since the early 1990s and is licensed up to 63 days gestation. Similar methods of achieving uterine evacuation have been developed for early miscarriage. Regimens use PG analogues, usually preceded by the antiprogesterone mifepristone. Success rates (i.e. total avoidance of surgery) is achieved in 95–98% of cases. Thirteen and a half thousand medical terminations were undertaken <9 weeks in 2000. Forty percent of NHS cases were dealt with medically but only 4% of cases managed by other purchasers. RCTs show high efficacy and acceptability, with a reduced incidence of pelvic infection compared to surgery. In this chapter, action plans are discussed for the management of complications associated with medically emptying the uterus in early/mid pregnancy.

CONSULT OTHER TOPICS

Complications of surgical management for therapeutic abortion and miscarriage (p 90)
Termination of pregnancy and maternal cardiac disease (p 101)
Therapeutic abortion – indications and the Abortion Act (p 87)
Upper tract pelvic infection (p 13)

Early medical termination/medical evacuation of the uterus

The regimens used for evacuation of the uterus for miscarriage and therapeutic abortion are very similar. When mifepristone is used, the priming dose of 200 mg is given 36–48 hours before PG analogues. Various regimens are described using different types, dosages and routes of administration for PG analogues. The main complications to consider are: abortion/miscarriage in the priming phase, heavy bleeding or collapse, no products of conception (POC) passed/failed medical methods and infection. These will be reviewed in the following mini-action plans.
NOTE: The action plans can also be applied to these complications when they occur during spontaneous miscarriage.

ABORTION/MISCARRIAGE IN THE PRIMING PHASE

MINI-ACTION PLAN

This occurs in <5% of cases of early medical abortion, but may complicate up to 30% of cases of 'missed miscarriage' managed medically.

1 **Discuss the possibility when mifepristone is given**
- Advise contact number.
- Admission recommended if 'heavy' bleeding +/– significant pain.
- Offer 'open access' to ward.

2 **Admission with bleeding +/– significant pain**
- If collapsed (rare) – institute ABCs of resuscitation (see haemorrhage below).

- Speculum examination – remove visible POC from vagina or open cervical os.
- If POC removed or tissue passed – start PG analogue. Examples to consider:
  a Oral misoprostol 400 μg stat and 200 μg 2 hours later.
  b Gemeprost 1 mg PV or misoprostol 800 μg PV.
- If POC not passed, defer PG treatment until 36–48 hours after mifepristone:
  a *Missed miscarriage* – oral misoprostol 600/400/400 μg at 2 hour intervals.
  b *Therapeutic abortion* – gemeprost 1 mg PV or misoprostol 800 μg PV.

3 **Do not forget to check Kleihauer and administer anti-D immunoglobulin in Rhesus-negative women**

HEAVY BLEEDING OR COLLAPSE WITH MEDICAL METHODS

Significant haemorrhage complicates <2% of procedures. Women who spontaneously miscarry may present in a similar way and require identical management.

1 **If collapsed – institute ABCs of resuscitation**

2 **iv access – send blood for FBC, group and save (X-match if appropriate)**

3 **Speculum examination**
- Remove blood clots/POC with a swab held in sponge-holding (ring) forceps.
- Visualize cervix.
- Remove any POC from within the cervical canal.

4 **Consider ergometrine 500 μg im or iv if bleeding continues**

5 **Thereafter, further heavy bleeding needs *URGENT* surgical uterine evacuation**
- Evacuation must not take low priority on a list – haemorrhage is a true emergency.

6 **Do not forget to check Kleihauer and administer anti-D immunoglobulin in Rhesus-negative women**

SUPPLEMENTARY INFORMATION

Speculum examination

Signs of collapse will be due to one of two causes: (1) vasovagal shock – related to POC trapped in a dilated cervix; (2) excessive haemorrhage. Although speculum examination will be fairly uncomfortable, IT IS MANDATORY when the patient is haemodynamically unstable, 'shocked' or bleeding heavily – explain this to the patient. The vagina can hide a significant amount of blood and blood clot. POC may or may not be contained within the clot (examine later). You may have to remove the speculum and digitally evacuate the blood clot from the vagina. The cervix should be visualized and POC within the canal removed. Again, this can be achieved digitally if speculum visualization is difficult.

NO POC PASSED AND FAILED MEDICAL METHODS

Medical methods result in complete evacuation in >95% of early abortions and miscarriages. True 'failure' of early therapeutic medical abortion (i.e. viable pregnancy after treatment) is rare (<0.5%). It is the responsibility of medical staff to ensure that the abortion process has occurred.

1 **No POC confirmed within 4–6 hours of PG analogue**
- Therapeutic medical abortion.
  a Occurs in 5% cases (final ongoing pregnancy rate will be much less**).
  b Discharge home with appointment for review in 7–10 days.
  c Pregnancy test/scan at review.
  d Arrange surgical abortion if still viable (<0.5%**).
- Missed miscarriage
  a May wish to consider surgical evacuation prior to discharge home.
  b Otherwise discharge home with appointment for review in 7–10 days.
  c Pregnancy test/scan at review.
  d Surgical evacuation only if sac still intact or 'excessive' bleeding.

2 **Do not forget to check Kleihauer and administer anti-D immunoglobulin in Rhesus-negative women**

INFECTION

Medical approaches to uterine evacuation are associated with a reduced risk of subsequent pelvic infection (0.3%) compared to surgery. However, chlamydial screening has been recommended for *all* women undergoing therapeutic abortion. Patients with post-abortal or post-miscarriage secondary infection, usually present with increasing bleeding (+/– lower abdominal pain) 7–10 days after the primary procedure. This usually implies underlying 'endometritis' and does not usually require surgical evacuation. Indeed, the more familiar the practitioner with medical methods, the less the subsequent intervention rates.

1 **General examination**

2 **Pelvic examination (including speculum)**
- Take appropriate swabs from endocervix (incl. chlamydia).

3 **Send bloods for FBC, group and save, (blood cultures if temperature >38°C)**

4 **Start broad spectrum antibiotics**
- Oral or iv dependent on clinical condition.

- If condition allows, review after 12–24 h of antibiotic therapy.
- Discharge home if bleeding settling with oral antibiotic course.
- Otherwise arrange ultrasound scan.

5 **Pelvic ultrasound scan**
- Heterogenous shadows may imply retained products, decidua or blood clot.
- Surgical evacuation if AP diameter >15 mm or if significant bleeding continues.
- In this circumstance, an experienced operator should perform the evacuation.

6 **Check chlamydial swab result**
- When reported, will need contact tracing and specific antibiotics if positive.

Midtrimester medical techniques

For the majority of practicing gynaecologists in the UK, medical techniques using combinations of antiprogesterone and PG analogues offer the safest approach to management of midtrimester abortion or intrauterine death (IUD). Mifepristone 200 mg halves the time required for PG to cause abortion or uterine evacuation. Various regimens are described and involve multiple doses of oral or vaginal PG analogue. Examples are: (a) misoprostol 800 μg PV then 400 μg orally 3 hourly (maximum four doses); (b) gemeprost 1 mg PV 3 hourly (maximum five pessaries). Fetocide with intracardiac 15% potassium chloride should be undertaken for medical abortions >21 weeks. This action plan reviews complications associated with midtrimester medical abortion/evacuation.

ACTION PLAN

1 **Consider prior screening for chlamydial infection**

2 **Confirm gestation by ultrasound scan**

3 **Oral mifepristone 200 mg 36–48 hours before PG analogue**

4 **Bleeding during 'priming` phase**
- Very infrequent with *midtrimester abortion*.
- May occur in up to 10% of *midtrimester IUD* managed medically.
- Usually defer PG until 36–48 h after mifepristone.
- If os open – start PG regimen earlier.

5 **Haemorrhage during PG administration**
- Establish iv access etc.
- Usually indicates passage of fetus +/– placenta.
- SPECULUM examination stat – fetus/placenta will be in cervix or upper vagina and can be removed with sponge-holding (ring) forceps.
- Give im or iv ergometrine 500 μg.

6 **Delay in passage of placenta**
- Fetus and placenta usually deliver together.
- If delay and no excess bleeding, continue PG if course is not complete.
- Speculum 4 h later – remove placenta if visible.
- Otherwise surgical evacuation (only 5–10% will need this).

7 **Failure to abort/miscarry within 24 h**
- Unusual in *IUD* and only reported in 4% of *midtrimester abortions.*
- *Repeat course of PG analogue (starting 24 h after start of first course).*

8 **Rare complications**
- Uterine rupture.
  a ↑ risk when process takes >24 h.
  b Suspect with risk factors (previous uterine scar, grand multipara).
  c Severe pain, haemodynamic instability.
  d Rupture may be posterior.
- Cervical tear.
  a ↑ risk when process takes >24 h.
  b May be 'silent'.
- Rarely these complications and intractable haemorrhage can lead to hysterectomy.

9 **Always remember to check Kleihauer and administer anti-D immunoglobulin in Rhesus-negative women**

REFERENCES

Abortion Statistics Annual Reference volume – Series AB 27 (2001). Legal abortions carried out under the 1967 Abortion Act in England & Wales, 2000. ONS, London. www.statistics.gov.uk

RCOG 'Greentop' guideline No. 11 (1997) *Induced abortion*. RCOG, London.

Hinshaw K and Fayyad A (2000) *The management of early pregnancy loss*. RCOG 'Greentop' guideline No 25. RCOG, London.

TERMINATION OF PREGNANCY AND MATERNAL CARDIAC DISEASE

Kate Grady and Kim Hinshaw

In the 1994–1996 Confidential Enquiry into Maternal Deaths (CEMD), 39 of the indirect deaths were due to cardiac disease. Ten of these were in congenital cardiac conditions and 29 in acquired conditions. Cardiac disease can be adversely affected in a predictable way by pregnancy or can worsen unexpectedly. Of the maternal deaths in those with congenital cardiac disease, six were due to primary pulmonary hypertension which worsens predictably. Three of these deaths were related to termination (one of these may have been related to pulmonary embolus). Other congenital cardiac causes were hypertrophic obstructive cardiomyopathy, aortic valve disease with endocarditis and anomalous coronary arteries. Antibiotic prophylaxis is important in the presence of valvular disease or a prosthesis. Acquired cardiac causes of death include myocardial infarction, cardiomyopathy, thrombosed mitral valve and pericarditis.

Joint cardiological and gynaecological assessment and investigation is necessary to quantify the risk of continuing pregnancy in a patient with a known cardiac condition. Termination may be justified under provision A of the Abortion Act (i.e. continuing pregnancy carries significant risk to the woman's life). Women with non-life threatening cardiac disease may of course request termination for psychosocial reasons (provisions C and D).

ACTION PLAN

1 **Consider diseases with serious risk associated with ongoing pregnancy**
   Major risk of complications or death.
   - Pulmonary hypertension.
   - Eisenmenger's syndrome.
   - Coarctation of the aorta (complicated).
   - Marfan's syndrome with aortic involvement.

2 **Consider implications of other cardiovascular disease in conjunction with cardiologist**

3 **If termination is proposed – consider relative benefits of surgical and medical methods**

4 **If surgical termination is proposed – involve consultant anaesthetist**

5 **With valvular disease or prosthetic valves – endocarditis is common**
   - Accounts for 10% of maternal cardiac deaths.
   - Use appropriate antibiotic prophylaxis.

6 **Refer to specialist centre as appropriate for those with *severe* heart disease who choose to continue with pregnancy**

CONSULT OTHER TOPICS

Complications of medical management for therapeutic abortion and miscarriage (p 96)
Complications of surgical management for therapeutic abortion and miscarriage (p 90)
Myocardial infarction (p 254)

Pre-operative investigation and fitness for anaesthesia (p 204)
Peri-operative management of common pre-existing diseases (p 208)

SUPPLEMENTARY INFORMATION

Consider diseases with serious risk associated with ongoing pregnancy

These categories are a guide only. In reality combinations of lesions and effects occur. Furthermore, lesions can be of varying severity. Cardiological investigation and the opinion of the cardiologist in each case is a more accurate guide to severity of disease and therefore risk. The management of ongoing pregnancy in these conditions is outside the remit of this text. The joint obstetric/cardiology assessment may conclude that termination of pregnancy is the safest option, but the final decision must remain with the pregnant woman.

Pulmonary hypertension •

One of the key recommendations in the CEMD states that 'pulmonary hypertension is very dangerous and requires careful management'. Pulmonary hypertension in pregnancy carries a grave prognosis. Due to the fall in systemic vascular resistance, the right to left shunt is allowed to increase so blood by-passes the lungs resulting in profound hypoxaemia. If there is a fall in systemic blood pressure there can be a dramatic fall in perfusion of the high resistance pulmonary circulation causing further hypoxaemia. Pulmonary hypertension is less likely to result from an atrial septal defect (ASD) than it is from a ventricular septal defect (VSD) or patent ductus arteriosus (PDA). Because of the high mortality associated with continuing pregnancy, termination is advised for the patient with significant pulmonary hypertension of any cause. The degree of pulmonary hypertension can be quantified by pulmonary artery catheterization.

Eisenmenger's syndrome

The syndrome develops when, in the presence of a left to right shunt, progressive pulmonary hypertension leads to shunt reversal or bi-directional shunting. Maternal mortality is reported as 30–50%. There is a reported 34% mortality with vaginal delivery and 75% associated with caesarean section. Eisenmenger's with VSD has a higher mortality than with ASD or PDA.

Coarctation of the aorta (complicated)

In coarctation of the aorta, the risk of death approaches 15% in the presence of aortic or intervertebral aneurysm, known aneurysm of the circle of Willis or associated cardiac lesions (VSD and PDA). Therapeutic termination should be considered.

Marfan's syndrome

Marfan's syndrome is an autosomal dominant disorder with connective tissue, skeletal, ocular and cardiovascular abnormalities (mitral or aortic regurgitation). The increased risk of maternal mortality during pregnancy is caused by involvement of the aortic wall which may result in aneurysm, rupture or dissection. The prognosis must be individualized by echocardiography. Patients with an abnormal aortic valve or aortic dilatation have up to a 50% pregnancy associated mortality.

Consider implications of other cardiovascular disease in conjunction with cardiologist

Moderate risk of complications

- Mitral stenosis with atrial fibrillation (if anticoagulated with heparin).
- Artificial valve (if anticoagulated with heparin).
- Mitral stenosis with severe functional limitation.
- Aortic stenosis.
- Coarctation of the aorta (uncomplicated).
- Uncorrected tetralogy of Fallot.
- Previous myocardial infarction.

Minimal risk of complications or death

- ASD or VSD (if anticoagulated with heparin).
- PDA (if anticoagulated with heparin).
- Pulmonary/tricuspid disease.
- Corrected tetralogy of Fallot. •
- Bioprosthetic valve.
- Mitral stenosis with limited functional impairment.
- Marfan's syndrome with normal aorta.

The physiological changes which occur and the way in which they can affect cardiac disease are as follows:

a In pregnancy there is an increase by 50% of circulating blood volume. If there is intrinsic myocardial dysfunction (low ejection fraction on echocardiogram), valvular disease or myocardial ischaemia, the increased volume may be poorly tolerated. This may cause congestive cardiac failure or myocardial ischaemia may be worsened because of the increased cardiac workload.

b Systemic vascular resistance (SVR) is reduced. In patients with the potential for right to left shunts, the shunt will be increased because of the fall in SVR (e.g. ASD, VSD and PDA).

c There is a need for anticoagulation in those with artificial valves and some with atrial fibrillation because of the hypercoagulable state of pregnancy.

d There are marked fluctuations of cardiac output particularly during labour. The potential for fall in pre-load as in vena caval obstruction or haemorrhage presents a serious risk to those dependent on adequate pre-load (i.e. those with pulmonary hypertension and fixed cardiac output as in mitral stenosis).

If termination is proposed – consider relative benefits of surgical and medical methods

Surgical abortion

The procedure is often carried out under local anaesthesia in other countries, but this is not common practice in the United Kingdom. This option may be considered in cases of severe maternal disease, but the involvement and presence of a consultant anaesthetist is recommended.

Medical abortion

Involves treatment with antiprogesterone followed 36–48 hours later by PG. When first introduced, PGs administered by im injection (e.g. 'Sulprostone`) were associated with several reports of sudden maternal death. This was usually in women over 35 years who were heavy smokers. Proposed mechanisms included coronary artery spasm, severe hypotension and ventricular arrhythmia. Prostaglandin E causes vasodilatation, with potential fall in systemic and pulmonary vascular resistance and resulting fall in blood pressure. The PGs used for therapeutic termination in first and second trimester are analogues of PGE_1, usually administered vaginally (gemeprost and misoprostol). The procedure is safe with few reports of significant complications. However, there are isolated reports of myocardial ischaemia induced by use of gemeprost in abortion. Care may be required if larger doses are used (e.g. midtrimester medical termination).

The relative risks of general anaesthesia/surgery vs. use of PG in medical termination must be assessed on an individual basis.

If surgical termination is proposed – involve consultant anaesthetist

Anaesthetic management should be in the hands of a consultant anaesthetist who should be given adequate notice to assess the patient. Depending on the seriousness of the condition, the anaesthetist may wish to refer the patient to a cardiothoracic surgery centre for operation.

FURTHER READING

Clark SL, Cotton DD, Hankins GDV and Phelan JP (1997) Cardiac disease. In: *Critical Care in Obstetrics*. Blackwell Science, Oxford.

Why mothers die. Report on confidential enquiries into maternal deaths in the United Kingdom 1994–1996. HMSO, London 1998.

ACUTE AND EMERGENCY MANAGEMENT OF MOLAR PREGNANCY

Steven Adair and Kim Hinshaw

Gestational trophoblastic disease (GTD) is classified by the WHO as follows:

- Hydatidiform mole – complete (CHM)   Pre-malignant
- Hydatidiform mole – partial (PHM)   Pre-malignant
- Invasive mole   Malignant
- Choriocarcinoma   Malignant
- Placental site trophoblastic tumour (PSTT)   Malignant

The last three are grouped together under the category 'gestational trophoblastic tumours' (GTTs). GTD is rare in the UK with an incidence of 1.54 per 1000 live births. It does occur more commonly in many parts of Asia, Africa and Latin America. CHM occurs more commonly in women <16 years or >40 years. The incidence of PHM is not related to age at conception. There is an increased risk of hydatidiform mole in women with a previous molar pregnancy.

- Previous CHM x 1 Risk = 1/76
- Previous CHM x 2 Risk = 1/6.5

COMPLETE HYDATIDIFORM MOLE

CHM usually presents earlier than PHM with first trimester bleeding (threatened or complete miscarriage). Often a 'large-for-dates' uterus is palpated and this may be filled with a bulky mass; the classical scan appearance looks like a 'bunch of grapes' (i.e. multiple sonolucent cystic areas of variable size – approximately 5–25 mm diameter). Presentation may be as a result of the very high hCG levels: hyperemesis, theca luteal cysts, hyperthyroidism or severe pre-eclampsia. Rarely, presentation is with severe haemorrhage. CHMs have the potential to develop into invasive moles. Also, women with pregnancies complicated by CHMs are at significant risk of developing choriocarcinoma (2–3%) or PSTT.

PARTIAL HYDATIDIFORM MOLE

In a PHM, there may be a co-existing fetus. There is an increased risk of TRIPLOIDY in the fetus. PHMs have been shown to develop into invasive moles, but there is NO evidence to show that they develop into choriocarcinoma or PSTT.

This chapter deals with the management of uterine evacuation for molar disease.

1 Suction curettage is the management of choice for evacuation of hydatidiform mole

2 Avoid medical uterine evacuation

3 iv access before procedure (two 16 gauge cannulae)

4 X-match blood available – 4 units

5 Avoid cervical preparation with prostaglandin

6 Suction curettage – can usually be achieved with 12 mm curette for evacuating CHM

7 In PHM the size of fetal parts may not allow the use of suction curettage. This is the *only* situation in which 'medical therapy' should be used routinely in primary management

8 If excessive bleeding at surgery, recheck cavity with suction curette. Use bimanual uterine massage and compression initially to encourage myometrial contraction

9 Use oxytocic infusion AFTER evacuation (20–40 units oxytocin in 1l N Saline at 250 ml/h)

10 Use prostaglandin analogues ONLY if oxytocic ineffective

11 If significant bleeding occurs before evacuation, oxytocin infusion may be required *during* the procedure

CONSULT OTHER TOPICS

Complications of surgical management for therapeutic abortion and miscarriage (p 90)

Scan findings relevant to the Early Pregnancy Assessment Unit (p 68)

SUPPLEMENTARY INFORMATION

Action points 2, 5, 9, 10

Oxytocics and prostaglandin analogues should be avoided prior to or during curettage because of the risk of intravascular dissemination.

Use PG analogues ONLY if oxytocic ineffective

Suitable PG analogues include gemeprost 1 mg or misoprostol 800 µg administered into the posterior vaginal fornix. In the presence of heavy vaginal bleeding, the vaginal route may be ineffective: consider RECTAL misoprostol 400–800 µg or prostaglandin F2α 250 µg (deep IM).

FURTHER READING

RCOG (1999) *The management of gestational trophoblastic disease*. RCOG 'Greentop' guideline. Royal College of Obstetricians and Gynaecologists, London.

PREGNANCY WITH AN INTRAUTERINE CONTRACEPTIVE DEVICE PRESENT

Kim Hinshaw

The intrauterine contraceptive device (IUCD) is a highly effective form of reversible contraception with a reported failure rate of 0.4–2.4 per 100 woman years. The presence of an IUCD is associated with an increased risk of EP. This association may be due to its excellent ability to prevent intrauterine pregnancy, rather than an actual increase in the number of EPs. This chapter deals with the management of intrauterine pregnancy with the IUCD *in situ*. Eighty percent of IUCD failures are related to incorrect placement. The failures also include cases of expulsion, perforation (partial or complete), and rarely translocation (i.e. spontaneous migration through the uterine wall – 0.2%).

Presentation may be to the early pregnancy unit, in gynaecology or antenatal clinics and occassionally as an emergency to the gynaecology ward.

ACTION PLAN

1 **Review history**
- What type of IUCD inserted?
- Any history of acute pain on insertion?
- When were the IUCD threads last checked?
- Has the IUCD location been checked previously by ultrasound?
- Is patient aware of IUCD expulsion?
- Consider possibility of EP.

2 **General and abdominal examination**

3 **Pelvic examination**
- Take swabs.
- Note presence or absence of IUCD thread.
- Is IUCD itself visible?

4 **Confirm patient's plans for the pregnancy**

5 **Ultrasound assessment**

6 **Removal of IUCD**
- Direct removal.
- Use of IUCD removal device (e.g. 'Emmet' thread retriever).
- Removal under ultrasound control.

7 **IUCD not located or not removed – subsequent management**
- X-ray of pelvis and abdomen if IUCD not confirmed at end of pregnancy.

CONSULT OTHER TOPICS

Complications of the intrauterine contraceptive device (p 42)
Ectopic pregnancy (p 76)
Scan findings relevant to the Early Pregnancy Assessment Unit (p 68)
Upper tract pelvic infection (p 13)

SUPPLEMENTARY INFORMATION

General and abdominal examination

With a confirmed pregnancy in the presence of an IUCD, history and examination should first aim to exclude the possibility of EP. Particularly consider this possibility in those cases admitted on an emergency basis with pain and bleeding. Look for localizing signs of lower abdominal pain or tenderness.

Pelvic examination

If undertaken prior to ultrasound assessment, the aim should be to note the presence or absence of the IUCD threads and to take appropriate swabs (including chlamydia). Removal is only recommended prior to scanning *if the end of the IUCD itself is visible* in the cervical canal or at the external os. This implies that the device is only partially in the cavity and below the gestational sac. It may still be prudent to confirm or refute viability in this circumstance before attempting removal.

Confirm patient's plans for pregnancy

Although an effective form of contraception was being used, many women with an unexpected intrauterine pregnancy will not wish to undergo termination. If termination is requested, take appropriate endocervical swabs (including chlamydia) and remove IUCD if thread accessible (see below). If thread not seen – arrange scan to confirm IUCD is *in utero*. This can be removed at the time of surgical abortion. If medical termination requested, IUCD must be sought in any tissue passed. Advise patient that surgical removal may be required if IUCD is not passed.

Women presenting with bleeding to the EPAU will be particularly concerned that IUCD removal may lead to miscarriage. There is a risk of miscarriage related to removal, but the risks are *HIGHER* if the IUCD is left *in situ*.

Ultrasound assessment

In early pregnancy, both TA and TV routes may be required. The following should be recorded:

- Confirmation of intrauterine pregnancy/viability/gestation.
- Presence of IUCD. The majority of IUCDs in use today are copper-based and easily visible on scan as they produce strong acoustic echoes. Progesterone-coated coils do not produce as strong acoustic shadows. If not visualized, the most likely diagnosis is expulsion. A coil that has completely translocated into the peritoneal cavity may not be seen on ultrasound because of gas in the bowel. X-ray may be required at the end of pregnancy to confirm (see below).
- Location of IUCD. Careful assessment in two scan planes is required to confirm position: inside the uterus, partially perforating the uterine wall, extrauterine, in cervical canal. For an IUCD which is in the uterus, its position relative to the pregnancy sac should also be noted.

Removal of IUCD

In the presence of a viable intrauterine pregnancy, IUCD removal in the first trimester should be offered. There is a higher risk of miscarriage if the IUCD is left *in situ*. The main risk of miscarriage is in the midtrimester and there is a striking association with intrauterine/fetal infection with *Candida* species. There is an increased risk of neonatal pneumonia or skin infection.

Direct removal

If the IUCD thread is easily visible, a careful attempt at removal should be made by pulling with ovum forceps or an artery clamp. The traction used should be *gentle and intermittent* which has been described as leading to successful extraction without gestation sac damage. If the thread is not visible, the cervical canal can be carefully explored with an artery clamp or plastic 'Emmet' thread retriever.

Use of IUCD removal device (e.g. 'Emmet' thread retriever)

Without ultrasound this should only be used to try and retrieve a thread *in the cervical canal.*

Removal under ultrasound control

Can be used for all removals or reserved for those cases when an attempt without scan control has been unsuccessful. In addition it may help removal in cases when the thread is not visible. It can be used with a hook specifically designed for IUCD removal.

IUCD not located or not removed – subsequent management

If the device is not seen on scan and the woman cannot definitely confirm expulsion, the IUCD must be sought at the time of miscarriage, termination or delivery. It will often be found morbidly adherent to the placenta or membranes. If not found, arrange X-ray of pelvis and abdomen to exclude the possibility of translocation (X-ray should include pelvic outlet and diaphragm on both sides).

FURTHER READING

Ranzini AC, Wapner RJ and Davis GH (1995) Ultrasonographically guided intrauterine contraceptive device removal before chorionic villus sampling. *Am. J. Obstet. Gynecol.* **173(2):** 603–605.

Shavel J, Greif M, Ben-Rafael Z, Itzchak Y and Serr DM (1982) Continuous sonographic monitoring of IUD extraction during pregnancy: preliminary report. *Am. J. Roentgenol.* **139(3):** 521–523.

Whyte RK, Hussain Z and deSa D (1982) Antenatal infections with *Candida* species. *Arch. Dis. Child.* **57(7):** 528–535.

LAPAROSCOPY

Christopher Mann, Jeremy Wright and Charles Cox

PROBLEMS WITH INSUFFLATION

The majority of gynaecologists use a Verres needle to achieve a pneumoperitoneum. General surgeons have adopted the open Hasson technique which they claim to be safer. Occasional surgeons introduce the primary trocar directly.

Failure to induce pneumoperitoneum with the Verres needle

ACTION PLAN

1 Suspect

2 Remove the needle and check that there is free flow of gas through it and that it is long enough

3 Palpate the abdomen

4 Make another attempt placing the needle through the thinnest part of the abdomen i.e. through the umbilicus

5 If unsuccessful consider the suprapubic approach

6 If still unsuccessful consider passing the needle through the posterior fornix or through the fundus of the uterus

7 Consider Palmer's point or the ninth intercostal space

8 Carry out open laparoscopy (Hasson's technique)

SUPPLEMENTARY INFORMATION

- Suspect that there is a problem if the pressure remains high or goes above the pressure set for the abdomen, or if the abdomen feels doughy and does not distend evenly. The abdomen should be hyper-resonant to percussion. Usually the diagnosis is made by passing the trocar and failing to reach the peritoneal cavity due to extraperitoneal gas.
- Remove the needle to check that it has not become blocked for example with patient's tissue. The tubing should have been checked before starting the procedure but check it again now and check that the insufflation machine is working.
- Palpate the abdomen to check for distension and previously unsuspected masses.
- Retry passing the Verres needle, it is not helpful to tent the abdomen by lifting up the abdominal wall. Attempt to place the needle through the thinnest part of the abdomen i.e. where the peritoneum is in contact with the posterior surface of the umbilicus.
- If unsuccessful at the umbilicus consider insufflating through a suprapubic approach, be careful to stick to the midline and do not angle the needle towards the head so as to reduce the risk of vascular damage.

- If still unsuccessful, consider passing the needle through the fundus of the uterus or through the posterior fornix of the vagina, especially in obese women.
- Insufflation has been carried out via Palmer's point 4 cm below the costal margin in the line of the nipple.
- The ninth intercostal space has also been described.
- The Hasson open laparoscopy is the preferred method of the surgeons and involves an incision below the umbilicus down to the peritoneum which is opened under direct vision. The main disadvantage to this procedure is cosmetic.
- Evidence at present does not suggest that open laparoscopy is necessarily safer than the use of a Verres needle and is certainly less cosmetic. It has been suggested that bowel injuries occur with the same frequency with both techniques but major vessel damage is less likely with the open method.
- A recent review of 350 000 laparoscopies reveals a rate of bowel damage during entry to be 0.4 per 1000 and the rate of major vessel injury to be 0.2 per 1000. These results are from so called centres of excellence and therefore may be an underestimate or vice versa! Animal work does not support the view that bowel damage is reduced by an open approach. There may be a benefit in producing a high intra abdominal pressure before introducing the trocar.

REFERENCE

Garry R (2000) Safe entry techniques. *Gynaecol. Endoscopy* **9 (suppl. 1):** 21.

GAS EMBOLISM

The inadvertent placement of a Verres' needle into a blood vessel may lead to a large volume of carbon dioxide entering the venous circulation and into the right side of the heart. Blood may be forced out of the heart by the gas and the remaining blood will become foamy. Cardiac output from the right side of the heart will cease and there will be circulatory collapse. The mortality rate associated with gas embolus is 40–50%.

<table>
<tr><td rowspan="6">ACTION PLAN</td><td>1</td><td>Suspect</td></tr>
<tr><td>2</td><td>Summon immediate senior anaesthetic and medical help</td></tr>
<tr><td>3</td><td>Remove the Verres needle and deflate the abdomen</td></tr>
<tr><td>4</td><td>Place the patient in the left lateral Trendelenburg position</td></tr>
<tr><td>5</td><td>Aspiration of gas from the right side of the heart should be attempted</td></tr>
<tr><td>6</td><td>The laparoscopic procedure should be abandoned</td></tr>
</table>

SUPPLEMENTARY INFORMATION

Suspicion of direct passage of gas into the circulation is suggested by the following findings:

- Circulatory collapse in the absence of massive blood loss.
- The presence of a loud murmur on cardiac auscultation (the cog-wheel murmur).

The patient should be placed on their left side and the legs elevated in order to encourage the gas to pass into the lungs (100% oxygen should be administered).

Aspiration of gas from the heart can be achieved by the passage of a central venous line into the heart and will be performed by an anaesthetist.

LARGE VESSEL TRAUMA

This may occur during placement of the Verres needle, the primary port or the lateral ports. The signs of circulatory collapse may be misinterpreted by the anaesthetist in the absence of any obvious blood loss. Iliac vessel injury may also occur during the placement of lateral ports which may be initially misplaced retro-peritoneally. Again, the bleeding may be disguised.

ACTION PLAN

1 **Suspect**

2 **Call for specialist senior surgical help**

3 **Immediately perform a laparotomy through a long lower midline incision**

4 **On entering the abdomen. Apply direct pressure to the bleeding site**

5 **Compress the aorta with your hand just above the bifurcation**

6 **Await specialist help**

SUPPLEMENTARY INFORMATION

- Suspect if there is circulatory collapse or a frank haemoperitoneum. Inspect the abdomen for obvious retroperitoneal haematoma or pelvic side-wall swelling.
- Vascular damage is particularly common in young patients with scaphoid abdomens or where there is devarication of the recti. A rapid explosive passage of the trocar especially if the trocar is felt to hit solid bone is also a worry!
- The vessels most commonly damaged are the right external iliac artery, aorta and vena cava.
- Damage occurring at placement of the primary port may not be immediately recognized as there may be initial vessel spasm, followed by rapid retro-peritoneal blood loss which may be obscured by overlying bowel.
- **The presence of an experienced vascular surgeon is essential. If it is apparent that a great vessel is transfixed leave the trocar in place as this will help tamponade the flow.**
- Place the patient in a steep Trendelenberg and make the incision with the scalpel that is provided with the laparoscopy instrumentation rather than waiting for a full laparotomy kit. Apply direct pressure to bleeding site – this may involve several large packs.
- Aortic compression just above the bifurcation will dramatically reduce blood flow while waiting for vascular expertise to arrive.
- Aorto-caval compression requires considerable pressure and surgeons should take turns in applying this. Having controlled the bleeding by aorto-caval compression it is better to wait for the appropriate help to arrive than to attempt repair oneself.
- **The long term sequelae of a major vessel injury such as claudication, reduced exercise tolerance or a 'heavy leg' can be avoided by appropriate and skilled vascular surgery.**

INFERIOR EPIGASTRIC VESSEL INJURY

The placement of lateral ports too medially, i.e. in the angle bordered by the obliterated hypogastric and the insertion of the round ligament into the anterior abdominal wall may result in damage to the inferior epigastric vessels. This may be arterial or venous and results in brisk bleeding from the port site and blood is seen to run down the trocar.

ACTION PLAN

1 **Suspect**

2 **Insert a second port on the contralateral side of the abdomen**

3 **Consider diathermy**

4 **Consider suturing**

5 **Pass a Foley catheter down the port track, inflate the balloon and apply traction**

6 **The port site incision may need to be extended and the vessels exposed to achieve haemostasis**

7 **A decision will need to be made with regard to continuing with the intended procedure**

SUPPLEMENTARY INFORMATION

- The diagnosis will usually be obvious with blood running down the trocar or a haematoma developing although the problem may not become apparent until the completion of the procedure due to the tamponading effect of the trocar.
- A bipolar forcep may be passed through the contralateral port. If the port on the bleeding side is plastic, it may be possible to diathermize the damaged vessel. If the port is metal, this will have to be removed prior to attempting to arrest the haemorrhage with bipolar diathermy.
- An attempt to suture the haemorrhage by a combined laparoscopic and external approach may be made.
- Pass a black silk suture on a long hand-needle through the abdominal wall lateral to the damaged port site. Pick this up and pass it back out of the abdomen medial to the port, so that both ends of the stitch are external. Tie tightly over a small gauze swab and observe the port site for further haemorrhage.
- If bleeding continues, pass a Foley catheter down the port site, inflate the balloon and apply traction. This is an extremely simple and efficient technique.
- If the bleeding is still not controlled explore the site by increasing the size of the port site incision. It may be difficult to expose vessels because of haematoma.
- A decision about whether or not to continue the procedure should be made in conjunction with the anaesthetist depending on the extent of the surgery and the condition of the patient.

VENOUS PELVIC SIDE-WALL BLEEDING

1 **Suspect**

2 **Avoid the blind use of diathermy**

3 **Apply pressure**

4 **Use lavage**

5 **Leave a drain**

SUPPLEMENTARY INFORMATION

- Dissection of adhesions on the side-wall may result in significant venous side-wall bleeding close to the great vessels.
- Application of indiscriminate diathermy to these may cause increased bleeding or damage to the great vessels and significant retro-peritoneal haemorrhage.
- The usual surgical principles of pressure apply although this is more difficult to maintain at laparoscopy. Pressure to the site should be applied with a sucker or other instrument and steadily maintained for at least 2 minutes by the clock.
- Following withdrawal of pressure the site may be observed with lavage but should not be palpated again for fear of starting bleeding.
- Leave a redivac or other drain adjacent to the oozing or original site of haemorrhage.

BOWEL INJURY CAUSED BY THE VERRES' NEEDLE

Inadvertent bowel injury with the Verres' needle may be of no consequence and is often unrecognized at the time of surgery. If recognized it can be managed with careful post-operative observation of the patient.

ACTION PLAN

1 **Suspect**

2 **Inspect**

3 **Lavage**

4 **Further observation**

5 **Administer a broadspectrum antibiotic**

6 **Decide whether a laparotomy is required**

7 **If so consider consulting a general surgeon**

SUPPLEMENTARY INFORMATION

- If gas flow has not been free and the needle has had to be inserted more than once then there is increased likelihood of bowel damage.
- If a large amount of gas has passed into the bowel prior to the injury being recognized, this may escape from the bowel together with liquid faecal content as a spray, causing widespread peritoneal contamination. Liberal lavage should be carried out with warmed saline until it runs clear. If there is an obvious breach of the bowel it may be worth putting in a laparoscopic suture if the operator is sufficiently experienced.
- Before being discharged the patient should be warned to report any increasing pain or gastro-intestinal symptoms directly to the gynaecological ward so that the operating surgeon can be informed. Patients who have had a laparoscopic procedure should get better quickly!
- Particular attention should be paid to the clinical signs of tachycardia, pyrexia and peritonism.
- Drainage of the abdomen is not usually necessary.

BOWEL INJURY CAUSED BY INSERTION OF THE PRIMARY TROCAR

Following insertion of the primary trocar insertion of the laparoscope will show intestinal mucosa demonstrating that a bowel perforation has occurred, alternatively the trocar may lacerate or transfix bowel especially if adhesions are present.

ACTION PLAN

1 **Suspect**

2 **Call for appropriate help**

3 **Leave the laparoscope and trocar in place**

4 **Extend the umbilical port incision along the length of the laparoscope in order to guide the operator to the area of perforation**

SUPPLEMENTARY INFORMATION

- Place a stay suture either side of the perforation and then withdraw the laparoscope.
- Repair the perforation in one or two layers.
- Check the other side of the bowel for an occult further perforation and inspect the rest of the bowel in case multiple loops of bowel have been damaged.
- It is rarely, if ever, necessary to defunction the bowel.

PERFORATION OF THE STOMACH

This is more common in patients with 'J' shaped stomachs and with the increasing use of laryngeal masks, as considerable volumes of gas may enter the stomach at this time. It is also more common when Palmer's point is used for insufflation. Preoxygenation also inflates the stomach, this may be detected by a fullness in the epigastrium.

ACTION PLAN

1 **Suspect**

2 **Ask for a naso-gastric tube to be passed before continuing with the procedure**

3 **Inspect the external anterior aspect of the stomach**

4 **Insert suture if necessary**

SUPPLEMENTARY INFORMATION

- Suspect from the appearance of the stomach mucosa. A naso-gastric tube seen in the stomach is diagnostic and one should be passed.
- It is not usually necessary to suture the stomach.

INADVERTENT ENTEROTOMY DURING A THERAPEUTIC PROCEDURE

Adhesiolysis, particularly of dense post-operative adhesions, may result in inadvertent enterotomy. These require immediate closure which can either be undertaken laparoscopically or at laparotomy, depending on the experience of the surgeon.

ACTION PLAN

1 **Suspect**

2 **Identify**

3 **Close**

4 **Consider drainage**

Careful observation and copious lavage may aid in the identification of bowel damage which is particularly likely to happen during surgery for endometriosis especially when dealing with disease in the recto-vaginal septum.

It may be possible to deal with bowel damage without laparotomy and it is rarely necessary to perform a colostomy.

Laparoscopy

URINARY TRACT DAMAGE

Damage to the bladder is more likely if the bladder is full. Perforation of the bladder with the Verres needle is unlikely to require any active treatment. Very occasionally there may be a patent urachus which may communicate with the bladder. The ureters are at risk during pelvic wall surgery for endometriosis or pelvic node dissection. If damage to the ureter is suspected the ureter should be catheterized and if this confirms a problem urological help should be requested.

ACTION PLAN

1 **Suspect**

2 **Catheterize the ureters**

3 **Request expert assistance**

BOWEL DAMAGE – POST-OPERATIVE PRESENTATION

Bowel damage at laparotomy is usually recognized and treated immediately whereas that at laparoscopy is usually delayed, leading to significant complications and morbidity. The guiding principles should be that recovery following a laparoscopic procedure should be smooth and steady.

Most patients undergoing laparoscopy are very fit and will maintain reasonable pulse and blood pressure despite worsening peritonitis until they finally collapse. Their care is frequently left to junior doctors or they are seen as emergencies following day case surgery and discharged home with analgesia, only to be admitted, moribund, 48 hours later. Any undue pain or discomfort post laparoscopy should be taken seriously. Patients should get rapidly better after laparoscopy. The following are all signs which may indicate intra-abdominal sepsis and should NOT be ignored:

- Tachycardia.
- Peritonism.
- Rising white cell count.

ACTION PLAN

1 **Contact the original operating surgeon and discuss the level of complexity of the procedure**

2 **Call appropriate surgical help**

3 **Arrange for urgent laparotomy and inspection**

4 **Resuscitate actively with fluids and antibiotics**

5 **Remember that faecal peritonitis carries a 25% mortality rate and that patients frequently require extensive stays in ICU with multisystem failure, repeat laparotomies and recurrent obstruction. Early recourse to laparotomy and suturing of defects is associated with an excellent prognosis**

INTESTINAL OBSTRUCTION

Herniae through port sites

ACTION PLAN

1 **Suspect**
2 **Consult a general surgeon early**

SUPPLEMENTARY INFORMATION

- The quoted incidence of post laparoscopy incisional hernia is 21 per 100 000 from a postal questionnaire sent to members of the American Association of Gynaecologic Laparoscopists.
- Herniae may be through the umbilical site or through the operative trocar sites.
- These may occur immediately after surgery with coughing during recovery from anaesthesia or in the immediate recovery period. Other herniae develop later.
- Omentum may herniate even through 5 mm ports and even if attempts have been made to close the defect. More seriously bowel may herniate through or partial thickness of the bowel may herniate into the larger port sites. If a loop of bowel herniates through the port site intestinal obstruction will rapidly develop. A Richter's hernia is more difficult to diagnose as the patient tends to have variable symptoms over several days because the obstruction is partial as only a part of the bowel wall is involved. It is however important to diagnose the condition reasonably early to avoid the bowel becoming non-viable and resection becoming necessary.
- Intestinal obstruction may occur from internal herniae, adhesions or kinking of the bowel in the absence of abdominal herniae.

REFERENCE

Montz FR, Holschineider CH and Munro MG (1994) Incisional hernia following laparoscopy: a survey of the American Association of Gynecologic Laparoscopists. *Obstet. Gynaecol.* **84:** 881–884.

HAEMORRHAGE – POST-OPERATIVELY

ACTION PLAN

1 Suspect

2 Resuscitate

3 Stop the bleeding

SUPPLEMENTARY INFORMATION

Haemorrhage may present with excessive blood loss through a drain although it should be remembered that drains get blocked! Big mistakes are made with little drains and small mistakes with big drains.

If the patient shows signs of haemorrhage investigation is required. If the patient is stable a laparoscopy can be carried out as a diagnostic and possibly therapeutic procedure. If the patient is shocked laparotomy is a better option.

Note: Laparoscopic mishaps are likely to be subject to critical incident inquiries and are increasingly the subject of medical litigation. In these circumstances concise, accurate, timed and dated notes will be invaluable in the defence of the operating surgeon.

Laparoscopy

HYSTEROSCOPY

Charles Cox

UTERINE PERFORATION

Usually occurs at the time of insertion. Women with a tight cervix (nullipara or those who have had cervical surgery with resulting stenosis) and women with acutely anteverted or retroverted uteruses are at greatest risk. Reduce risk of perforation by bimanual examination and inserting the scope under direct vision.

Perforation at the time of insertion

ACTION PLAN

1 Consider a laparoscopy especially if the patient has had previous pelvic surgery and you suspect that bowel may be stuck to the uterus

2 Observe the patient for a few hours

3 Consider the use of prophylactic antibiotics

Perforation at the time of an intrauterine procedure (especially if diathermy was being used)

ACTION PLAN

1 Carry out laparoscopy

2 Examine bowel for evidence of a burn or other damage, evidence of thermal damage to the bowel carries a high risk of subsequent perforation often delayed for a few days

3 Examine pelvic side walls for damage to blood vessels or ureters

4 If there is active bleeding it may be possible to deal with this laparoscopically but if in doubt carry out a laparotomy through a midline incision. If you require assistance from the surgeons you can be sure that they will want to make the incision bigger!

5 Whilst waiting for assistance control haemorrhage by direct pressure. Direct compression of the aorta may be necessary in the case of major vessel damage

6 Consult senior colleague or other appropriate specialities

7 Observe patient post-operatively especially if an open operation has not been carried out

8 Administer prophylactic antibiotics

FLUID ABSORPTION

Large amounts of absorbed glycine used as a distension medium for endometrial ablation or resection can lead to dilutional hyponatraemia. This may lead to potentially fatal complications such as intravascular haemolysis, hepato-renal failure and cerebral oedema. Fluid discrepancy should be monitored carefully and if more than 1000 ml of glycine is unaccounted for the procedure should be terminated and consideration given to the administration of diuretics. A urinary catheter should be put in place.

A sodium level of 120 mmol/l is a critical level for serious reactions. ECG changes occur at 115 mmol/l. Fitting occurs at 102 mmol/l and at levels below 100 mmol/l ventricular tachycardia or fibrillation can occur.

There may be a delay in recovering from the anaesthetic; if under regional or local anaesthesia confusion and coma may occur.

ACTION PLAN

1 **Suspect**

2 **Monitor fluid absorption**

3 **Be especially vigilant with patients who have heart disease**

4 **Stop the procedure when 1000 ml of fluid is unaccounted for**

5 **Measure the sodium level**

6 **If the sodium level is below 120 mmol/l consider the use of intravenous hypertonic saline and diuretics**

7 **Mannitol 10–20% may be used as an osmotic diuretic and does not cause further hyponatraemia. It is also said to be more effective at reducing cerebral oedema**

SUPPLEMENTARY INFORMATION

- Fluid in and out should be checked at 10 minute intervals.
- Fluid may be absorbed directly and rapidly into the blood stream when vessels are cut across as in endometrial resection and care must be taken not to have too much pressure on the fluid going into the uterus.
- A reasonable pressure is between systolic and diastolic pressure.

HAEMORRHAGE – PRIMARY AND SECONDARY

- This may be primary or secondary.
- It is unusual after ablation or resection but more common after resection of fibroids.

Primary haemorrhage

ACTION PLAN

1 Rollerball obvious bleeding areas

2 Be careful when dealing with persistent bleeding at the ostia because the uterus is at its thinnest and at greatest risk of perforation

3 Insert a Foley catheter with a 20 ml balloon or bigger and inflate it

4 Leave for at least 4 hours and up to 24 hours

5 Do not forget that bleeding can come from the Vulsellum forceps on the cervix and can require suturing

Secondary haemorrhage

Classically occurs 10–14 days after the procedure and may resolve with antibiotics. Heavier bleeding may respond to the insertion of a Foley catheter.

ACTION PLAN

1 Insert a Foley catheter into the uterus and inflate the balloon

2 Administer broad spectrum antibiotics

3 Consider exploration of the uterus to remove necrotic debris

INFECTION

If a focus of infection is present the procedure should not be carried out as there is a risk of severe sepsis.

Prophylactic antibiotics are not mandatory although commonly given.

ACTION PLAN

1 **Take vaginal swabs, if the patient is pyrexial take a blood culture**

2 **Commence broad spectrum antibiotics**

3 **Organize an ultrasound scan in due course to check for a pelvic collection**

FURTHER READING

The MISTLETOE study of endometrial resection shows a low mortality and a 1% rate of emergency surgery including laparoscopy, laparotomy, and hysterectomy.

Overton C, Hargreaves J and Maresh M (1997) A national study of complications of endometrial destruction for endometrial disorders: the MISTLETOE study. *Br. J. Obst. Gynaecol.* **104**: 1351–1359.

HYSTERECTOMY

Paul Hooper

PROBLEMS OF ACCESS

At abdominal hysterectomy

1 A vertical incision is recommended with any large pelvic mass. Extension of the vertical incision, or an inverted 'T' incision to a transverse incision, can be used to improve access

2 Spend time on packing and arranging the retractors

3 A two-staged removal of the uterine body, and subsequent removal of the cervical stump, may improve access if a large fibroid uterus is present or there are dense adhesions

4 If access is very difficult it may well be safer to carry out a subtotal hysterectomy which will reduce the risk of damage to the urinary tract and also to the rectum if stuck to the back of the cervix

5 Use the myomectomy screw to apply traction to the uterus

6 Ensure adequate lighting and assistance

7 Request assistance early

At vaginal hysterectomy

1 When you obtain consent for vaginal hysterectomy discuss the possibility of conversion to an open procedure

2 Do assess vaginal capacity and access

3 Check uterine size, mobility and descent

4 Preliminary laparoscopy may be helpful in assessing suitability for the vaginal route

5 The impression of prolapse is often given by cervical hypertrophy and elongation and patience will be needed to take the pedicles a step at a time. Do not be afraid to take multiple small pedicles and to ligate them as you go

6 Do not be afraid of bisecting the uterus to allow access to the upper pedicle

7 Techniques such as myomectomy may make the procedure simpler and placing the myomectomy screw in a largish fibroid improves access and makes it easier to deliver the uterus

8 An early decision to convert to an abdominal route must be considered in cases of difficult access or excessive bleeding

PRIMARY HAEMORRHAGE

1 Direct pressure to the bleeding area with a gauze swab will 'buy time' to assemble clamps, sutures and suction, and to also consider surrounding structures and tissues. Accurate placement of an appropriate clamp will often stop bleeding, but before placing sutures around the clamp, there should be a careful check to exclude bladder, bowel or ureter from the sutured area

2 When the bleeding is of venous origin, direct pressure with a 'hot', i.e. just tolerable to skin, soaked pad may be sufficient to stop bleeding. Tissue sutures may be useful, but can sometimes cause further bleeding

3 Be careful of 'blind' clamping

4 Diathermy may be useful, but careful consideration must be given to the potential damage to surrounding tissues, particularly bowel and ureters, due to heat dissipation

5 Haemostatic matrix products may be applied to areas of venous oozing

6 If oozing persists, then consideration must be given to leaving an appropriate suction drain, or to leaving the vaginal vault open to facilitate drainage. Vaginal packing (with bladder catheterization) may be useful if bleeding is from vaginal skin edges

7 Failure of these initial measures to arrest bleeding should lead the surgeon to request senior assistance. Cross-matched blood should be ordered, and the anaesthetist informed of the excessive bleeding

8 If there is torrential bleeding, manual occlusion of the aorta or vena cava should be considered, whilst a vascular surgeon is summoned. Ligation of either or both internal iliac arteries may be required to control bleeding. Consideration should also be given to pelvic packing, which is removed at a second laparotomy, or to arterial embolization

Hysterectomy

DAMAGE TO BOWEL

The most likely time to damage bowel is when opening the abdomen. Many lacerations may be dealt with by simple suturing. It is very important however not to narrow the bowel and the patency should be checked by grasping the lumen between the finger and the thumb.

ACTION PLAN

1 **Examine the length of the bowel if damage is suspected**

2 **Check whether the bowel is viable**

3 **Check on the blood supply, there should be bleeding from the edges and the bowel should be pink. If in any doubt consult a surgeon**

4 **If bowel is to be resected check the arterial arcades**

5 **Close the mesentery when anastomosis is complete**

6 **Insert a naso-gastric tube**

Colostomy

The possibility of a colostomy should be discussed if surgery is being carried out for malignant disease or severe degrees of pelvic sepsis e.g. actino-mycosis or severe endometriosis.

ACTION PLAN

1 **If contemplating a colostomy seek senior advice**

2 **A loop colostomy is the simplest procedure and is a temporary measure**

3 **A suitable place is in the upper abdomen in the midline where a transverse incision is made, the transverse colon drawn out and a rod placed underneath the bowel. The bowel is opened on its anti-mesenteric border through a taenia**

4 **The left iliac fossa may be used as long as no further surgery is planned in that area**

Hysterectomy

POST-OPERATIVE HAEMORRHAGE

Reactionary haemorrhage usually occurs 4–6 h after surgery (but up to 24 h), and may be caused by sub-optimal management of primary haemorrhage, a rise in post-operative blood pressure, ligature slippage, or removal of primary clot following coughing or movement. It may be visible, as bleeding from the wound, vagina or as excessive loss in drainage bottles, but should be suspected if the patient becomes restless, clammy and cold with an increasing pulse rate.

If bleeding from the vagina

ACTION PLAN

1 Resuscitation should be commenced whilst making arrangements to return to theatre to rectify the problem. Remember that the surgery is part of the resuscitation and do not allow time to be taken up trying to restore the patient's blood pressure and pulse to normal before taking the patient to theatre

2 If there is obvious bleeding from the vagina put the patient in the lithotomy position and consider bleeding from the angle of the vagina. Insert sutures as appropriate. Pack and catheterize

3 If bleeding not controllable from below open the old incision

4 Have adequate suction and plenty of packs

Secondary haemorrhage

Secondary haemorrhage occurs 7–14 days following surgery, and is usually thought to be due to infection.

ACTION PLAN

1 Assess – does the patient require an operative procedure?

2 If bleeding from the vagina do a speculum examination to check for active bleeding. If oozing from the vault the vagina may be packed, a catheter inserted and antibiotics started

3 Resuscitation should be undertaken, and appropriate bacteriological investigations taken prior to commencing broad spectrum antibiotics

4 Vault haematoma formation with subsequent infection is easily identified at vaginal examination, when gentle probing can often achieve drainage of the haematoma

5 Abdominal wall haematomas, particularly those underlying the rectus sheath, may be harder to identify clinically, but may be detected by ultrasound at which time drainage of the haematoma may be indicated

6 Superficial wound haematomas often discharge spontaneously, when the sinus may be enlarged to facilitate drainage

INFECTION

1 **Suspect**

2 **Identify likely site**

3 **Use appropriate broad spectrum antibiotic**

4 **Consider drainage**

SUPPLEMENTARY INFORMATION

- Antibiotic prophylaxis should be considered in all patients undergoing hysterectomy.
- Urinary tract infection is the most common cause for post-operative pyrexia. It is relatively easy to diagnose, and rarely causes difficulty in diagnosis or management.
- Post-operative pneumonia, however, may be difficult to differentiate from pulmonary embolus. It should be suspected in any patient with breathlessness, pyrexia or cough, particularly in smokers. Chest physiotherapy and antibiotics are the mainstay of treatment. Specialized investigations such as VQ scans and ultrasound may be required.
- Wound infections are easily identified clinically, and appropriate bacteriological specimens should be obtained prior to antibiotic therapy. Superficial infections rarely cause serious complications, but infection with *Streptococcus pyogenes* or *Clostridium perfringens* can cause severe necrosis extending into underlying muscle, and should be suspected if rapidly spreading necrotizing tissue is seen around the wound site. Antibiotic treatment should be guided by a microbiologist, and excision of necrotic tissue should be undertaken immediately.
- Where there is pus, let it out.

WOUND DEHISCENCE

Wound dehiscence is a rare complication that may follow infection, but can occur due to poor closure technique.

ACTION PLAN

1 **The exposed abdominal contents should be covered with saline soaked swabs and arrangements made for theatre**

2 **Debridement of infected areas should be followed by resuturing with non-absorbable sutures in a mass closure**

3 **Antibiotics should be started and adequate drainage of the wound ensured**

SUPPLEMENTARY INFORMATION

Later problems include wound sinus formation which is usually secondary to foreign materials.

Wound sinus

ACTION PLAN

1 **Explore and excise the tract and remove any foreign material, usually a suture**

2 **Close the wound if you are sure that the tract has been excised and it is not actively infected**

3 **Otherwise allow the tract to granulate. A pack may be necessary to keep the wound open while healing occurs to prevent reformation of the sinus tract**

Hysterectomy

PROBLEMS WITH DRAINS

Drains are usually inserted in cases of continued haemorrhage or to protect suture lines in the bowel or urinary tract. Small drains do not always drain!

If the drain is not draining consider withdrawing the drain a little and flushing it through.

Continued drainage of large volumes of fresh blood, suggest ongoing bleeding. Laparotomy is usually indicated, but techniques such as arterial embolization may be appropriate. The presence of fluid resembling urine may indicate damage to the urinary tract. An IVU should be arranged, and if extravasation of urine is confirmed, the case should be discussed with a urologist.

Removal of drains may sometimes be difficult. This may be due to inadvertent inclusion of the drain in the closure sutures, or may be due to the position of the drain. Indiscriminate and excessive traction on drain tubes is extremely uncomfortable and may result in snapping of the drain with subsequent difficulty in retrieval. Re-exploration and removal of the drain should be carried out in theatre.

URINARY TRACT DAMAGE

The development of vaginal leaking of urine, presence of urine in drainage bottles, or the development of unilateral (or bilateral) loin pain should raise the possibility of urinary tract damage.

ACTION PLAN

1 **Suspect**

2 **Examine the patient and carry out simple investigations**

3 **Request radiological investigations**

4 **Consult a urologist**

SUPPLEMENTARY INFORMATION

- Do not diagnose stress or urge incontinence in post-operative patients who did not have these conditions before.
- A bedside speculum examination should be carried out and a catheter placed in the bladder and dye instilled into it.
- An intravenous urogram should be carried out. A vesico/uretero-vaginal fistula may be difficult to identify on IVU. A triple swab test using methylene blue instilled into the bladder may help in reaching a diagnosis. Obstruction of either ureter will lead to hydronephrosis and delayed emptying on IVU. Percutaneous nephrostomy is usually performed to relieve hydrostatic pressure prior to definitive management by the urologists.

OTHER COMPLICATIONS

OGILVIE'S SYNDROME

Ogilvie's syndrome (pseudo-obstruction) may complicate hysterectomy. It is more common in elderly patients, and those with renal or cardiac problems, who are confined to bed. There is increasing abdominal distension, often dramatic, with bowel sounds which may become obstructive in character. Water-soluble contrast enemas may establish the absence of mechanical obstruction, and colonoscopy may be used to diagnose the condition and to decompress the colon. Management is usually conservative with intravenous nutrition and correction of electrolyte abnormalities.

HERNIA

Herniae, either internal or through the abdominal wall, can lead to mechanical obstruction and a Richters hernia where part of the bowel wall is strangulated presents more slowly with intermittent obstruction.

PSEUDO-MEMBRANOUS ENTEROCOLITIS

Pseudo-membranous enterocolitis is a complication of antibiotic therapy which presents with severe diarrhoea.

ILEUS

Paralytic ileus is common after abdominal surgery especially when there has been extensive handling of the bowel e.g. when bowel adhesions have been separated prior to definitive surgery or where bowel has been damaged.

Mechanical obstruction may result from kinking of the bowel or the formation of adhesions.

The patient will become distended. The differential diagnosis includes acute gastric distension, gastric dilatation and faecal impaction.

BOWEL COMPLICATIONS IN OTHER GYNAECOLOGICAL SURGERY

Charles Cox

The bowel is at risk of direct damage at the time of operation. Post-operative ileus is common and adhesions may develop post-operatively to cause intestinal obstruction. Occasionally pseudo-membranous colitis may develop as a reaction to antibiotics.

THE MANAGEMENT OF OPERATIVE INJURIES TO THE BOWEL

Most injuries to the bowel are avoidable. The riskiest time for the bowel is when the peritoneum is being opened. Other factors are haste to get on with the procedure and resulting lack of respect for the tissues with subsequent tearing and the injudicious use of clamps, retractors, haemostats and scissors. Lack of experience in handling bowel affected by adhesions, endometriosis, radiation, inflammation including TB or malignancy is also a major factor.

ACTION PLAN

1 **Suspect and inspect if concerned about bowel damage or bowel pathology**

2 **Carry out a systematic laparotomy**

3 **Inspect the small bowel from the duodenal-jejunal flexure to the terminal ileum**

4 **Inspect the stomach, firstly the anterior stomach and if the posterior surface of the stomach needs to be examined open the gastro-colic omentum to allow access**

5 **Pancreas and duodenum. The body and tail of the pancreas can be inspected by making a hole in the gastro-colic omentum. Further exposure of the pancreas and duodenum should be undertaken by a general surgeon if necessary and involves dissecting the hepatic flexure of the colon and transverse meso-colon off the pancreas distally and mobilizing the pylorus and gastric antrum caudally. The duodenum would need to be Kockerised to assess the posterior aspects of the duodenum and head of the pancreas**

6 **The colon and rectum. Inspect the ascending, transverse and decending colon and rectum. The ascending and descending colon and rectum are retroperitoneal and need to be mobilized for a full inspection of both anterior and posterior aspects**

7 **The liver, spleen and retroperitoneum should be checked**

8 **If a laceration to the bowel is identified a decision needs to be made whether to close the laceration or to resect the piece of damaged bowel. This decision depends on the viability of the bowel and whether it can be closed without narrowing it**

9 **Help should be sought from a general surgeon**

10 The viability of the bowel is judged by its colour, it should be pink not blue! The edges of the bowel should bleed freely when cut

11 If a decision to resect bowel is made the arterial arcades should be identified

12 Bowel may be closed by stapling, one or two layers of sutures or even by skin staples

13 The mesentery should be sutured to prevent internal herniae

14 The need to form an emergency colostomy should be infrequent and if is adjudged likely in the preoperative assessment consent should be explicitly obtained

15 A temporary loop colostomy can be brought out in the midline through a transverse incision above the umbilicus. The loop has a rod passed under it and the bowel is opened transversely along a taenia

16 Occasionally damage may occur to the sigmoid or rectum during difficult surgery for endometriosis or pelvic inflammation particularly actinomycosis. In this case a Hartmann's procedure may be carried out, bringing out a colostomy in the left iliac fossa and closing the distal colon or rectum

POST-OPERATIVE INTESTINAL OBSTRUCTION

Obstruction can occur after any intraperitoneal operation. Early adhesions are more likely to occur if there has been peritoneal irritation. Obstruction occurs when these adhesions kink the bowel. This is usually apparent in the first week after surgery. The common cause of apparent post-operative obstruction is of course paralytic ileus.

Paralytic ileus

Some degree of paralytic ileus is almost inevitable after any abdominal surgery and the more the bowel is handled and the more dissection there is around the bowel the more prolonged it is likely to be. The more significant degrees of ileus are usually noted between 48 and 72 hours.

ACTION PLAN

1 Treat post-operative nausea and vomiting

2 Listen to and palpate the abdomen. The abdomen is likely to be silent, distended and tympanic

3 Restrict diet and sometimes fluids especially if vomiting persists

4 If symptoms do not improve it may be necessary to pass a naso-gastric tube

5 If ileus is persistent especially if the patient is febrile a retained foreign body should be considered as should the rare complication of extravasation of urine

6 If ileus does not settle consider a mechanical obstruction and consult a surgeon

Suspected mechanical obstruction

ACTION PLAN

1 **Suspect. Paralytic ileus to some extent is normal after abdominal surgery but should be expected to improve over the first few post-operative days**

2 **If there is abdominal pain and vomiting an examination may show distension and hyperactive bowel sounds associated with the spasms of pain**

3 **If obstruction is suspected take plain films of the abdomen. Fluid levels on an erect film suggest obstruction**

4 **Post-operatively it is reasonable to treat obstruction with a naso-gastric tube. However, it should be remembered that there is a high rate of bowel ischaemia with small bowel obstruction and improvement should occur after a day or two**

5 **If not settling consult a surgeon**

OTHER BOWEL PROBLEMS ENCOUNTERED POST-OPERATIVELY

Acute gastric distension and dilatation

In acute gastric distension which is comparatively common after surgery large amount of air is swallowed leading to distension of the stomach which can even lead to splinting of the diaphragm.

ACTION PLAN

1 **A naso-gastric tube should be passed and left *in situ* until ileus has recovered**

Gastric dilatation is a serious post-operative complication with a mortality of up to 50%. The stomach distends with fluid and if not relieved secondary haemorrhage may occur into the stomach.

2 **Suspect if vomit contains brown or black material (altered blood)**

3 **Attend to fluid balance – large amounts of fluids and electrolytes will have been lost**

Faecal impaction leading to constipation and spurious diarrhoea

ACTION PLAN

1 If a patient develops diarrhoea post-operatively a rectal examination should be performed

2 If solid faeces are encountered the stool should be softened with glycerine suppositories or an oil retention enema and a digital evacuation of the rectum carried out

Pseudo-membranous colitis

ACTION PLAN

1 Suspect – if severe diarrhoea in a patient on antibiotics, due to an overgrowth of *Clostridium difficile*

2 Take a stool sample

3 Consider referral for emergency colonoscopy to detect pseudo membranous changes

4 Rehydrate the patient with particular care given to electrolyte balance

5 Commence vancomycin or metronidazole after consulting with the Microbiologists

The management of bowel obstruction in gynaecological patients with terminal malignant disease

ACTION PLAN

1 Administer steroids

SUPPLEMENTARY INFORMATION

There is a trend that corticosteroids of dose 6–16 mg dexamethasone given iv may bring about the resolution of bowel obstruction. Equally the incidence of side effects in all the included studies is extremely low. Corticosteroids do not seem to affect the length of survival of these patients.

REFERENCE

Feuer DJ and Broadley KE (2000) Cochrane Library Update Issue 4, Software Reviewers Conclusions.

ACUTE RETENTION OF URINE

Mamdouh Guirguis and Charles Cox

INTRODUCTION

Acute retention of urine is a condition seen predominantly in men and rarely in women. Patients with acute urinary retention present with severe discomfort and a sudden inability to pass urine, and the history and clinical findings quickly point to the diagnosis. However, in the presence of a neurological lesion or following an epidural anaesthetic it may be painless. The inability to void should be over 12 hours, requiring catheterization with removal of a volume equal to or greater than bladder capacity.

Herpes simplex is believed to be the most common cause of acute urinary retention in younger sexually active people, especially women. Acute retention can also be caused by post-operative pain, urethral oedema or immobility, a retroverted gravid uterus, urinary tract infection, urethral stricture, constipation and neurological disorders.

ACTION PLAN

1 **Suspect from history**

2 **Examination would show a full bladder, which may be tender, confirm by ultrasound if required**

3 **Analgesia for pain**

4 **Pass a self-retaining Foley's catheter for free drainage for around 1–2 days and send a catheter specimen of urine**

5 **Suprapubic catheter is required rarely if there is a urethral stricture (extremely rare in women although stenosis of the external urethral meatus can occur)**

6 **Once the catheter is removed, the voiding and residual volume of urine should be monitored**

SUPPLEMENTARY INFORMATION

Acute urinary retention associated with herpes simplex

It is often accompanied by systemic symptoms, constipation, inguinal lymphadenopathy, and local neurological disturbance, sometimes in the absence of clinically obvious herpetic lesions, which have been described as occurring up to 8 days after and 3 weeks before urinary retention occurred. Cervical or urethral herpetic lesions may be missed unless careful clinical examination is carried out.

For some patients it is sufficient to advise them to urinate in a warm bath; catheterization will be needed in less than a quarter of cases. In cases in which anogenital herpes is possible we advise that swabs should be taken and cultured for herpesvirus. After a clinical diagnosis, antiviral treatment should be started.

Acute urinary retention associated with postpartum epidural analgesia

This is not uncommon. Nursing or medical staff occasionally fail to enquire about voiding and painless retention develops. In neglected cases, up to 4 l of urine can be withdrawn. This produces a grossly overdistended bladder, which may fail to function and leave the patient with retention for up to 3 months or more. Some patients will have permanent voiding disorders.

CHRONIC RETENTION OF URINE

Mamdouh Guirguis and Charles Cox

INTRODUCTION

In women, outlet obstruction is rare but can occur in those who have had previous surgery for incontinence or who have a large cystocele that prolapses and kinks the urethra on straining to void.

Other causes include antispasmodic drugs, psychosis, and neurological or inflammatory conditions. Chronic urinary retention may result in overflow incontinence. Secondary detrusor over activity may also develop giving rise to urge incontinence.

Obstruction due to neurologic disease is invariably associated with a spinal cord lesion. Interruptions in pathways to the pontine micturition centre where outlet relaxation is coordinated with bladder contraction, cause detrusor-sphincter dyssynergia. Rather than relaxing when the bladder contracts, the outlet contracts, leading to severe outlet obstruction with severe trabeculation, diverticula, and a 'Christmas tree' deformation of the bladder; hydronephrosis; and possibly renal failure.

Chronic retention occasionally results from fusion of the labia minora in the elderly and may present with dribbling incontinence.

If the bladder is overstretched for any length of time then the detrusor muscle may not recover function immediately. Thus, a suprapubic catheterization (SPC) is more appropriate in patients with chronic retention so that 'trials without catheter' can be performed simply by clamping the catheter, which avoids repeated urethral catheterization if the patient fails to void successfully.

Catheterization may be followed by post-obstructive diuresis, and careful monitoring of urea and electrolytes concentrations and iv fluids may be needed. A chronically distended bladder does not need to be drained in stages as complications rarely ensue.

ACTION PLAN

1 **Suspect particularly following bladder neck surgery or if there is a large cystocele. A palpable, percussible and non-tender bladder is strongly suggestive**

2 **Diagnose by low flow rate on flowmetry, small voided volumes and large post-micturition residual volumes**

3 **Free drainage by self-retaining catheter for 1–2 days and then try to monitor voiding as described above. Send a CSU for culture and sensitivity**

4 **If there is outflow obstruction following tension-free vaginal tape, urethral dilation or division of the tape may be required**

5 **Voiding difficulties following colposuspension may require clean intermittent self-catheterization or a SPC**

6 **Management of the underlying cause, i.e. anterior repair**

SUPPLEMENTARY INFORMATION

Post-operative voiding difficulties

Black *et al.* (1997) have shown that up to 1 in 6 women reported difficulty urinating for up to 3 months after incontinence surgery, patients should be warned of this potential problem. Voiding should be closely monitored not only following incontinence surgery, but also following all kinds of pelvic surgery including Caesarian sections. It is important to make sure that the patient empties her bladder well by monitoring the voided volumes of urine and checking the residual urine if suspicion of incomplete emptying arises. Particular attention is given to those patients who had incontinence surgery. Following colposuspension, the SPC is usually left for free drainage for 2–3 days when it is clamped with continuous monitoring of the voided and residual volumes of urine. The SPC is usually removed as soon as satisfactory voiding with a minimal residual is achieved. The acceptable maximum residual is 100 ml.

Labial fusion may be managed by breaking down the adhesions under anaesthetic.

REFERENCE

Black N (1997) Impact of surgery for stress incontinence on morbidity: cohort study. *BMJ* **315:** 1493–1498.

HAEMATURIA

Mamdouh Guirguis and Charles Cox

Microscopic haematuria is defined by the detection of more than 5 RBCs/hpf or +ve dipstix test. Haematuria may be caused by any form of urinary tract pathology including carcinoma or it may be a post-operative finding. It may be difficult to know whether bleeding is coming from the vagina, the bladder or occasionally the bowel. The gynaecologist should therefore be prepared to carry out a competent cystoscopy as part of the investigation of post-menopausal bleeding.

If the patient presents with frank haematuria she should be referred to a urologist.

WHERE THE DIAGNOSIS OF HAEMATURIA IS NOT CLEAR

ACTION PLAN

1 **History and examination**

2 **Renal function tests**

3 **Urine microscopy and culture**

4 **Refer to urologist unless in menstruating women, UTI, suspected false positive or recent strenuous exercise when the urine should be tested again in around 1 months time**

5 **Cystoscopy and radiological imaging for diagnosis and treatment**

6 **Refer to nephrologist if there is proteinuria, red cell casts or renal impairment**

POST-OPERATIVE HAEMATURIA

ACTION PLAN

1 **Suspect possible bruising to or minor or major bladder injury depending on the kind of surgery**

2 **Measure urinary output, and observe the colour of urine**

3 **Usually draining the bladder by leaving the self-retaining catheter and antibiotics is all what is required**

4 **An intravenous urogram should be requested if ureteric damage is the suspected injury**

URINE LEAKAGE PER VAGINUM – FISTULAE

Mamdouh Guirguis and Charles Cox

Women with urinary fistulae (uretero-vaginal, vesico-vaginal, urethro-vaginal) often complain of uncontrollable, continuous urinary leakage, which usually occurs after pelvic surgery, advanced pelvic malignancy, or radiotherapy. A small recent fistula may heal spontaneously if urine is diverted from the fistulous tract. If a fistula is diagnosed within 48 hours of surgery, and if there is no major inflammatory reaction or necrosis about the fistula, immediate re-operation and repair should be considered. If inflammation is present then treatment should be interim continuous bladder drainage.

Continuous urinary leakage also appears to occur when the labia are fused. This may occur spontaneously due to oestrogen lack in the older woman, previous vulval surgery such as vulvectomy or uncommonly in this country as a sequelae of female circumcision. The urine is passed into the vagina which acts as a reservoir which leaks slowly away after micturition has been completed.

Vesico-vaginal fistula

Late recognition of bladder injury is common following gynaecological surgery. Most frequently the injury is found 5–14 days post-operatively when a clear vaginal discharge is noted. Hysterectomy associated bladder injuries classically appear between the ureteric orifices at the back of the trigone. These defects may be large, but usually are less than 1.5 cm in size, and do not usually involve the ureters. Other rare causes of vesico-vaginal fistula are obstetric injuries and following irradiation.

ACTION PLAN

1 **Suspect from history and finding urine in the vagina on speculum examination**

2 **Confirm by triple swab methylene blue test (The lower two sterile vaginal swabs stain blue following intravesical methylene blue dye instillation)**

3 **Cystoscopy to identify the site, size and extent of the fistula**

4 **Drain the bladder by a Foley's catheter for 2–4 weeks**

5 **Refer to a surgeon with the appropriate skills for a formal closure**

6 **Spontaneous fistula closure may happen during the waiting time if the fistula is very small**

7 **The traditional advice has been to wait for 2–3 months before surgery is performed for surgical fistulae and 6–12 months for post-irradiation fistulae. This is to allow inflammation to subside and for the tissues to become well vascularized. These days however it is not usual for patients to be prepared to wait so long after an initial trial of a catheter has failed**

Uretero-vaginal fistula

The venial sin is injury to the ureter but the mortal sin is failure of recognition. Unrecognized injuries associated with gynaecological surgery are responsible for the majority of these lesions. Radical hysterectomy, extensive pelvic surgery associated with malignancy, adhesions and/or endometriosis may be associated with an increased risk. Pelvic irradiation may rarely cause this kind of fistula.

ACTION PLAN

1 **Suspect from history and finding urine in the vagina on speculum examination**

2 **Exclude the possibility of either vesico-vaginal fistula or an associated vesico-vaginal fistula by triple swab methylene blue test (The lower two sterile vaginal swabs would not stain following intravesical methylene blue dye instillation)**

3 **Cystoscopy and examination under anaesthesia**

4 **Drain the bladder by a Foley's catheter for 2–4 weeks or proceed to closure**

5 **Intravenous urogram + delayed films (lateral and oblique)**

6 **Retrograde ureterogram**

7 **Refer to a surgeon with the appropriate skills for a formal closure**

8 **Spontaneous fistula closure may happen during the waiting time if the fistula is very small**

SUPPLEMENTARY INFORMATION

The waiting time before formal closure has traditionally been 2–3 months for surgical lesions and 6–12 months for post-irradiation fistulae, to allow for the inflammation to subside and for better vascularization. However, nowadays women are not prepared to wait these lengths of time and an attempt to close these socially disabling injuries is usually made shortly after recognition to reduce patient distress and litigation!

Urethro-vaginal fistula

This fistula may occur following a vaginal repair, surgery to, or infection of, a urethral diverticulum or obstetric trauma. It may also occur after irradiation.

ACTION PLAN

1 **Suspect**

2 **Urethroscopy, vaginoscopy, cystoscopy and examination under anaesthesia**

3 **A catheter may be inserted through the fistula to aid visualization**

4 **Drain the bladder by a Foley's catheter for 2–4 weeks**

5 **Retrograde urethrocystogram**

6 **Refer to a surgeon with the appropriate skills for a formal closure**

Vesico-uterine and uretero-uterine fistula

This type of fistula is rare now following improvements in obstetric practice. However, it is occasionally seen following a difficult caesarian section. It may be associated with cyclic haematuria and secondary amenorrhoea.

ACTION PLAN

1 **Suspect**

2 **Investigate**

3 **Consult a urological colleague**

4 **Repair with urological colleague**

SUPPLEMENTARY INFORMATION

Intermittent haematuria may occur coinciding with menses. An iv urogram is essential and cystoscopy and hysteroscopy may be helpful.

BLADDER INJURY IN GYNAECOLOGICAL SURGERY

Mamdouh Guirguis and Charles Cox

The bladder is relatively resistant to injury when collapsed and it usually moves away from the finger or scissors as it is not a fixed pelvic structure. When the bladder becomes fixed due to inflammation, cancer or previous surgery, the likelihood of bladder injury increases. Very thin bladder, loss of normal tissue planes and injudicious surgical dissection increase the risk of injury.

ACTION PLAN

1 Suspect in the presence of the predisposing factors and the appearance of wetness in the wound

2 Confirm by the instillation of methylene blue dye and filling the bladder

3 Define the extent of injury and the margins of lacerations by cystoscopy and the ureters catheterized to be sure that they have not been compromised by the injury and to protect them during repair

4 Immediate repair when discovered during gynaecological surgery

5 Refer to a surgeon with appropriate skills is recommended if the bladder tear is difficult, infected, devascularized or if the ureter is suspected to be involved

6 Closure of the bladder should be performed with 2–0 chromic or polygolic acid suture on a half-circle tapered needle. A simple running or running lock stitch placed in two layers will produce a secure closure

7 Following closure, the bladder should be filled to capacity to check for leaks

8 A figure-of-eight suture placed over the initial repair may be necessary to eliminate leaks

9 Cystoscopy may confirm bladder repair and the absence of ureteric involvement

10 Drain the bladder by a Foley's catheter for 7–10 days

11 Antibiotics for 7–10 days

URETERIC AND URETHRAL DAMAGE AT THE TIME OF GYNAECOLOGICAL SURGERY

Mamdouh Guirguis and Charles Cox

URETERIC INJURY

Ureteric injuries at the time of gynaecological surgery occur infrequently, with reported rates of 0.24–0.4%. Gynaecological disease often involves one or both ureters. Complex pelvic surgery and laparoscopic surgery may be associated with an even higher incidence. The reported incidence may be low, as many ureteric injuries are not recognized or reported. Ureteric injuries are the most common complication of gynaecological surgery leading to litigation, accounting for 17% of non-obstetrical legal actions initiated against obstetricians and gynaecologists.

- Ureteric injuries may occur at the pelvic brim, near the infundibulopelvic ligament, the pelvic sidewall, where the ureter passes beneath the uterine artery and at the vaginal fornix.
- Mechanisms of injury include inadvertent ligation, distortion or kinking, crushing, devascularization and compression from haematomas. Ureteric injury may also occur at the time of vaginal and abdominal procedures (open or laparoscopic) to correct stress urinary incontinence and pelvic floor prolapse.
- Although identification of the ureter at the time of surgery will reduce the incidence of ureteric injury, it will not entirely eliminate it. Such occurrences should not imply negligence. The ureter is particularly at risk in the presence of endometriosis, previous retroperitoneal dissection and adhesions, pelvic masses or procidentia. Some gynaecological surgeons routinely expose the ureter by retroperitoneal dissection during abdominal operations where adnexal surgery or hysterectomy is planned. There has been no prospective study of this method. A retrospective analysis by Neumann *et al.* showed a statistically significant reduction in ureteric injury following routine retroperitoneal dissection of the ureter.
- During pelvic surgery the surgeon must be conscious of the location of the ureters during every step of the procedure. During abdominal surgery, when the normal pelvic anatomy is distorted by disease, the surgeon should identify and trace the course of the ureter. During laparoscopic surgery, the same level of caution is recommended, with particular attention to the risks of cautery and stapling devices.

ACTION PLAN

1 **Prevention**

2 **Suspect**

3 **Identify the ureter**

4 **Repair**

SUPPLEMENTARY INFORMATION

Routine identification and tracing the course of the ureter is recommended during gynaecological surgery, including laparoscopic surgery involving the use of electrosurgery, laser and stapling devices. This may be performed through transperitoneal visualization, palpation or retroperitoneal dissection. The placement of ureteric stents pre-operatively has not been shown to decrease the risk of ureteric injuries. Although their use remains unproven in gynaecological surgery, the placement of stents may be considered in situations of high clinical concern.

When concern of possible injury exists verification of ureteric patency is recommended. Ureteric catheters may be passed via a cystoscopy. A cystotomy may be performed if necessary. Indigo carmine or methylene blue may be injected intravenously to identify the ureteric orifices and determine ureteric patency.

Immediate repair by a surgeon with appropriate skills is recommended when obstruction or damage is found intra-operatively. Uretero-vesical implantation is the method of repair if the ureter is divided near to the bladder. A Boari flap may be used if a portion of ureter adjacent to the bladder has been damaged otherwise a ureteric anastomosis should be carried out.

The maintenance of high clinical suspicion for ureteric injury following gynaecological surgery is recommended, with early investigations for definitive diagnosis. Patients complaining of flank pain or tenderness, especially in combination with fever or an ileus should have early investigation by ultrasonography and intravenous pyelography. Stanhope *et al.* observed a mean rise in serum creatinine of 71 μmol/l (range 27–24 μmol/l) at 36–48 hours post-operatively from pre-operative levels in patients with unilateral ureteric obstruction; so measuring pre- and post-operative creatinine levels may be useful. Appropriate referral may be necessary for management of ureteric injuries detected post-operatively.

URETHRAL INJURY

Injury to the urethra during vaginal or uterine surgery is very rare. More common is injury to the bladder neck, perforation of the bladder or fistula formation during urethral diverticulectomy.

ACTION PLAN

1 **Suspect and diagnose by cystoscopy**

2 **A urethrogram with double balloon technique or a nipple on a Foley catheter may be helpful in making the diagnosis**

3 **Prompt repair if the defect is fresh. Small defects may be closed primarily but large defects may require vaginal flap closure and interposition of a fat pad**

4 **Diversion of bladder urine with a SPC if the injury shows signs of inflammation**

REFERENCE

Neuman M, Eidelman A, Langer R, Golan A, Bukovsky I and Caspi E (1991) Iatrogenic injuries to the ureter during gynecologic and obstetric operations. *Surg. Gynecole Obstet.* **173:** 268–272.

Stanhope CR, Wilson TO, Utz WJ *et al* (1991) Suture entrapment and secondary ureteral obstruction. *Am. J. Obstet. Gynecol.* **164:** 1513–1517.

TRAUMA TO THE LOWER URINARY TRACT

Mamdouh Guirguis and Charles Cox

NON-SURGICAL BLADDER TRAUMA

- The bladder accounts for about 20% of external GU trauma.
- External bladder trauma is caused by blunt or penetrating trauma to the lower abdomen or pelvis, usually from RTAs or falls.
- Iatrogenic bladder injuries can result from endoscopy, laparoscopy or open pelvic surgery.
- Complications specific to bladder injury include infection, incontinence, and bladder instability.
- Mortality is about 20% and is related to the extent of associated injuries.

1 **Suspect if there is haematuria associated with any of the described type of trauma**

2 **Suggestive clinical findings include abdominal tenderness or distension, pelvic fracture, and inability to void**

3 **Cystography is used to confirm the diagnosis and classify the bladder trauma**
- Extraperitoneal ruptures are the most common type of major bladder trauma and are usually associated with pelvic fractures.
- Intraperitoneal ruptures involve the dome and usually occur with bladder distension at the time of trauma.
- Contusions represent damage to the bladder wall without urinary leakage and can result in medial bladder displacement.

4 **The choice of treatment depends on the type of bladder trauma and the extent of associated organ injuries**
- Extraperitoneal ruptures should be repaired surgically, unless they are small and do not involve the urinary sphincter mechanism at the bladder neck region. In such cases, a large transurethral catheter may provide sufficient drainage for healing.
- Intraperitoneal ruptures require prompt surgical exploration and repair.
- Bladder contusions can be managed with transurethral catheter drainage.

NON-SURGICAL URETERIC TRAUMA

- External ureteric trauma constitutes about 1% of all cases of GU trauma.
- Penetrating trauma from gunshot wounds is the most common cause.
- Overall, iatrogenic injuries are the most frequent causes of ureteric trauma and result from ureteroscopy, abdominal hysterectomy, or low anterior colonic resection.

- Complications of ureteric trauma include infection, fistula, and stricture. Early diagnosis of ureteric trauma and careful reconstruction of the ureter are important in minimizing complications and preserving renal function.

1 **A high index of suspicion is required because early symptoms and signs are not specific. Haematuria is absent in ≥ 30% of cases**

2 **IVU: If the results are inconclusive, retrograde ureteropyelography should be performed**

3 **Occasionally the diagnosis is made in the operating room during abdominal exploration. With delayed diagnosis, clinical findings include prolonged ileus, urinary leakage, urinary obstruction, anuria, and sepsis**

4 **Management depends on the elapsed time to diagnosis, the mechanism of injury, and the general condition of the patient**

5 **When the condition is immediately diagnosed, prompt surgical repair is the preferred treatment**

6 **In an unstable patient or when ureteral trauma is identified post-operatively, the first step is to insert a percutaneous nephrostomy tube to divert the urine. Imaging studies are then performed to further characterize the injury and plan appropriate surgical repair. Reconstructive techniques include ureteral reimplantation, primary ureteral anastomosis, anterior bladder flap, ileal interposition, and autotransplantation**

NON-SURGICAL URETHRAL TRAUMA

- External urethral trauma constitutes about 5% of GU injuries but is uncommon in women.
- Most major urethral trauma is due to blunt trauma.
- Penetrating urethral trauma is more common in women and may be associated with sexual assault.
- Iatrogenic injury occurs from endoscopy or catheter manipulation of the urethra. Potential complications of acute urethral trauma include stricture formation, infection, and incontinence.

1 **Suspect from a history of the described possible trauma**

2 **Before a urethral catheter is inserted, the meatus should be closely inspected. Blood at the urethral meatus is the best indicator of urethral trauma**

3 **Retrograde urethrography is used for diagnosis and classification: Contusions represent urethral stretching and do not cause extravasation of contrast. Partial disruptions result in periurethral extravasation, with some contrast entering the bladder. Complete disruptions are characterized by loss of urethral continuity and prevent filling of the bladder or proximal urethra**

4 Although urethral trauma often presents complex problems, a favorable outcome can be achieved with careful evaluation and appropriate management, which is chosen after the trauma is identified and accurately classified

5 Contusions can be safely treated with a 10 day course of transurethral Foley catheterization

6 Urethral disruption in women is very unusual. Suprapubic cystostomy drainage is the simplest option and can be used safely whilst consulting with regard to longer-term management

POST-OPERATIVE ANURIA

Mamdouh Guirguis and Charles Cox

If the patient does not pass urine several hours following surgery and, if an indwelling catheter is not already in use, a catheter is passed. A few millilitres of dark concentrate urine, possibly blood stained is obtained and the worst is immediately suspected. The possibilities are:

- Acute renal failure.
- Bilateral ureteric obstruction or obliteration.
- Bladder or urethral injury.
- Catheter problems.

ACTION PLAN

1 Check that the urethral catheter is inserted correctly and not obstructed. Flush the catheter with saline if obstructed

2 Suspect hypovolaemia or dehydration due to underestimated blood loss and treat by iv fluid replacement including blood transfusion and measure urine output. The suspicion is increased with difficult gynaecological surgery, low blood pressure, rapid pulse rate or with obvious postoperative haemorrhage. iv fluid replacement should produce immediate diuresis with an improved urine output. The use of CVP line may be indicated. Possible internal haemorrhage may require return to the operating theatre for haemostasis

3 Suspect bilateral ureteral obstruction or unilateral ureteral obstruction in a patient with one kidney due to congenital absence or previous nephrectomy should be raised if the catheter fails to produce any urine in the absence of hypovolaemia. Ureters can be clamped, ligated or severed in the course of a difficult operation for pelvic cancer. Rapidly deteriorating general condition of the patient, deteriorating renal function tests and ultrasound should be diagnostic

4 IVP and ascending urethro-cystography may be required

5 Immediate referral to renal physician and urologist

RENAL COLIC

Mamdouh Guirguis and Charles Cox

The symptoms resulting from renal and ureteric stones can be predicted from knowledge of the likely site of obstruction. Renal colic usually starts abruptly with flank pain, which then radiates around the abdomen as the stone progresses down the ureter. Typically pain is felt in the labia majora in female patients.

ACTION PLAN

1 **Suspect the diagnosis and provide adequate analgesia**

2 **Routine urine analysis (Some patients have frank haematuria, but the rest have microscopic haematuria, if the results of urine analysis are normal then an alternative diagnosis should be considered)**

3 **Intravenous urography unless they have a history of allergy to contrast media or are pregnant (renal ultrasonography is useful in these circumstances to show caliceal dilatation on the affected side)**

4 **Refer to urologist**

IMMEDIATE COMPLICATIONS OF OPERATIONS FOR URINARY INCONTINENCE

Mamdouh Guirguis and Charles Cox

COLPOSUSPENSION

Colposuspension is probably the gold standard operation for stress incontinence. Immediate complications are damage to the bladder, bleeding and unrecognized damage to the ureter.

Damage to the bladder

ACTION PLAN

1 Recognize the injury, consider placing dye in the bladder to give early warning of bladder damage

2 Repair the bladder with an absorbable suture in one or two layers

3 Drain the bladder for 5–10 days

4 Drain the retropubic space until catheter clamping is established.

Intra-operative bleeding

Bleeding is common from the veins in the cave of Retzius

ACTION PLAN

1 Do not immediately try to stop the bleeding especially with diathermy

2 If bleeding from deep down put a swab in and place the sutures in the vagina and ilio-pectineal ligament

3 If bleeding from the vagina the suspensory sutures may double as haemostatic sutures

4 Bleeding normally improves when the suspensory sutures are tied

5 Drain the retropubic space

6 Remember to take all the swabs out!

TENSION-FREE VAGINAL TAPE

Major complications have been infrequently reported to date but include haemorrhage, bladder perforation and rarely damage to the obturator nerve.

Haemorrhage – it is possible to go 'off line' while introducing the needle through the retropubic space and anecdotally major vessels have been damaged.

ACTION PLAN

1 Moderate bleeding can usually be controlled by a vaginal pack

2 More severe bleeding will require laparotomy with the availability of a vascular surgeon

Bladder perforation

This is not uncommon during passage of the needle and is rarely a long-term problem if recognized at the time.

ACTION PLAN

1 If the needle is detected in the bladder at cystoscopy the needle should be withdrawn and reinserted

2 If the needle continues to perforate the bladder on subsequent passes or there is significant loss of cystoscopic fluid vaginally the procedure should probably be abandoned for the present

3 The bladder should be drained with a catheter for a few days

Obturator nerve damage

Symptoms may arise if the needle goes 'off line' and comes into contact with the obturator nerve on the pelvic side-wall. If the patient is not under a GA she will draw this to your attention!

ACTION PLAN

1 Suspect

2 Draw the needle back and redirect it

3 Observe for haemorrhage

4 Hope that any neurological signs settle!

EMERGENCY PRESENTATIONS ASSOCIATED WITH PROLAPSE

Paul A. Moran

Acute urinary retention

This is usually secondary to a UTI, to which women with significant cystoceles are more prone as a result of 'stagnant urine' sitting within the prolapsed bladder base. Alternatively it may be due to urethral obstruction secondary to 'acute' kinking of the urethra (although this is more likely to present with chronic retention).

ACTION PLAN

1 Catheterize (suprapubic may be preferable)

2 Send urine for culture

3 Commence antibiotics (given likely cause)

4 Check urea and electrolytes

5 Insert a pessary to relieve obstruction or symptoms until definitive surgery can be performed

6 Exclude other causes e.g. a pelvic mass or a neurological problem

Chronic urinary retention

Chronic retention presenting with a UTI or secondary renal failure (which may present non-gynaecologically e.g. acute confusional state). This is usually as a consequence of urethral kinking/obstruction but may rarely (in gross prolapse) be due to bilateral ureteric obstruction.

ACTION PLAN

1 Suspect chronic retention as a cause of presentation

2 Suspect prolapse (e.g. large cystocele, vault prolapse, procidentia) as a cause of chronic retention and perform a vaginal examination

3 Exclude a pelvic mass

4 Catheterize, culture the urine, commence antibiotics and check renal function. If there is renal failure involve the renal physicians early and arrange renal ultrasound

5 Reduce the prolapse (this may require a GA if chronic and indurated)

6 Insert a shelf pessary

7 Await renal recovery before planning definitive surgery

Bleeding

Post-menopausal bleeding from decubitus ulceration

These ulcers occurs in large chronic prolapse (e.g. procidentia, vault eversion) and are secondary to tissue hypoxia as a consequence of gravitational oedema. They are always found on the most dependent part of the cervix. These ulcers are not malignant. Secondary infection and poor oestrogenization are common. It may rarely present acutely as fresh post-menopausal bleeding with a 'malignant looking' vaginal wall ulcer. In women with a uterus exclude endometrial malignancy.

ACTION PLAN

1 Suspect decubitus ulceration if the tissues are indurated and there is an everted prolapse found on examination

2 Swab the ulcer. Perform an endometrial biopsy if there is a procidentia (usually easy to do)

3 Send urine for culture and check the haemoglobin and electrolytes

4 Consider ultrasound to check endometrial thickness and residual urine

5 Commence antibiotics for secondary infection

6 Reduce the prolapse, under a general anaesthetic if necessary

7 Treat with local oestrogen. Healing of the ulcer will occur in a few weeks with local oestrogen treatment. Options include daily packing or placing an oestrogen-releasing ring pessary on top of a shelf pessary

8 Perform definitive surgery only when the ulceration and infection have resolved

VAGINAL EVISCERATION (BOWEL IN THE VAGINA)

Paul A. Moran

Vaginal evisceration is rare. It may occur spontaneously or secondary to rupture of a large enterocele and occasionally associated with malignancy of the genital tract. It is more likely to occur post-operatively after vaginal vault surgery.

It can also occur after vigorous intercourse where it is usually associated with oestrogen deficiency.

ACTION PLAN

1 **Resuscitate if necessary**

2 **Wrap eviscerated bowel in gauze soaked in saline. Arrange laparotomy**

3 **At laparotomy withdraw bowel through defect and inspect for mesenteric lacerations, bleeding and viability**

4 **Excise necrotic vaginal tissue and close the vaginal vault. Obliterate the cul de sac (e.g. Moschowitz procedure) if rupture has occurred through an enterocele**

5 **Anticipate ileus**

6 **Insert a naso-gastric tube**

7 **Cover the operation with antibiotics**

CONSULT OTHER TOPICS

Bowel complications in other gynaecological surgery (p 137)

SPECIFIC PERI-OPERATIVE COMPLICATIONS OF PROLAPSE SURGERY

Paul A. Moran

GENERAL COMPLICATIONS

Primary haemorrhage

At anterior colporrhaphy significant haemorrhage can occur from the rich venous plexus of the urogenital diaphragm.

Bleeding from broad tissue planes is common. A general ooze should not be ignored and may result in significant blood loss, delayed primary haemorrhage or haematoma formation.

ACTION PLAN

1 Small bleeding points on the vaginal mucosa, bladder and rectal muscle should be clamped and either tied or ligated

2 Bleeding from the vessels of the urogenital diaphram can be difficult to expose but can usually be controlled with figure-of-8 sutures

3 Pedicles at vaginal hysterectomy should be carefully ligated as slippage can result in a large primary haemorrhage. Transfixing the pedicles makes them less likely to slip

4 Traction should not be applied to sutures on vascular pedicles

5 Good access, retraction, light suction and capable assistance are essential

6 Laparotomy will be required if the bleeding point cannot be secured vaginally

Delayed primary haemorrhage (reactionary)

Persistence of fresh bleeding (through the pack and onto the bed!), particularly within the first 3 hours after surgery strongly suggests that haemostasis has not been secured!

ACTION PLAN

1 Resuscitate

2 Check blood count and haematocrit. Blood should be X-matched

3 Arrange an examination under anaesthetic

4 Examine the patient in the lithotomy position. Remove pack – use retractors, ensure good light and adequate assistance

5 Use long straight or Littlewood's forceps to provide traction on the vault

6 If there is bleeding from the suture lines use additional sutures to secure the bleeding points and repack for 24 h

7 If the bleeding is heavier with large clots, excessive bleeding or apical bleeding open the suture lines to try and identify bleeding source. Ligate or cauterize the bleeding points then close and repack. The common site for bleeding is from the vaginal angle and can usually be dealt with by a vaginal approach

8 Brisk bleeding from the vault after vaginal hysterectomy suggests that a large vessel has escaped its pedicle and is likely to be bleeding intra-abdominally. Pack the vagina for identification and proceed to laparoscopy or laparotomy depending upon the haemodynamic state of the patient and your experience with operative laparoscopy

Urinary tract injuries

Injuries to the urethra, bladder and ureter(s) are not uncommon, particularly in complex vault surgery, redo surgery and in the hands of an in-experienced operator.

ACTION PLAN

1 Suspect and recognize the problem. Routine cystoscopy would be appropriate after a complex or difficult procedure

2 At cystoscopy identify both ureters and wait for passage of urine down both. Diluted methylene blue dye may be instilled into the bladder if there are concerns about the integrity of the bladder

3 If a urinary tract injury is confirmed ask for senior help possibly a urologist, cover with antibiotics, explore the extent of damage, excise devitalized tissues and implement repair. Use absorbable sutures. Ensure that there is no tension at the repair site and employ bladder drainage for a minimum of 7 days

SITE SPECIFIC MANAGEMENT

Urethra

Can occur at anterior colporrhaphy, particularly in women who have had previous repair surgery. Usual injuries are stitch penetration or laceration. Proximal urethral laceration may damage the sphincter mechanism and lead to stress incontinence. There is a small long-term risk of developing a urethro-vaginal fistula.

1 Suspect

2 Perform a cystoscopic examination of the bladder and urethra using a zero degree cystoscope with a fine probe available

3 Remove the suture which has breached the urethra. It may be necessary to repair the urethra over a trans-urethral catheter with 3/0 or 4/0 absorbable suture

4 If it is suspected that the sphincter mechanism has been damaged buttressing of the bladder neck should be considered. More severe damage may require a Martius graft

5 Leave the catheter in 5–7 days

Bladder

Stitch penetration should be recognized either intra-operatively at cystoscopy or suggested by acute post-operative haematuria. If not dealt with there is a long-term risk of intractable cystitis and the formation of a stone or fistula. Laceration to the bladder resulting from surgical injury to the bladder during vaginal hysterectomy will occur almost exclusively in the area of the bladder base that is above and separate from the trigone and lower ureters. This is in contrast to tears at anterior colporrhaphy (i.e. upper third of anterior vaginal wall) where the ureters are at risk. There is a long-term risk of fistula formation after bladder damage especially if there is a poor blood supply e.g. after radiotherapy sepsis and if the defect has not been repaired in layers.

1 Carry out a cystoscopy

2 If the stitch is identified it should be removed. This can usually be carried out under cystoscopic control but may rarely require an open cystotomy

3 In the case of damage during vaginal hysterectomy the laceration is likely to be away from the trigone and the ureters. The defect should be closed, a cystoscopy carried out and the ureters identified and catheterized

4 If the bladder is damaged during anterior colporraphy damage is more likely to the ureters and in this case the ureters need to be cystoscopically identified and catheterized prior to repair. Repair should be in two layers with 2/0 or 3/0 absorbable suture and the bladder drained for a minimum of 7 days.

Ureteric damage

Damage may result as a consequence of kinking, suture entrapment, crushing and laceration. Have a high level of suspicion and perform cystoscopy after an extensive or difficult procedure and observe ureteric 'release'. If damage is suspected get senior urological assistance. Treatment options include simple suture release, ureteric stenting or ureteric re-inplantation if divided or badly damaged. Arrange follow-up iv urogram +/– a voiding cystogram to exclude stenosis or reflux.

Remember: Unilateral costo-vertebral tenderness associated with nausea occurring within 24 hours post-operatively in an afebrile patient is ureteric obstruction until proved otherwise – check for pyuria and arrange an urgent intravenous urogram.

Long-term risks if unrecognized are fistula formation, pyelonephritis and destruction of kidney.

ACTION PLAN

At the time of operation

1 Suspect – bleeding from the angles of the vagina which requires sutures to control, bleeding from the pelvic side-wall, dissection around the pelvic side wall and the presence of adhesions particularly from endometriosis that will distort the normal anatomy

2 Identify the ureter at the pelvic brim and trace it down to the bladder

3 If uncertain carry out a cystoscopy at the end of the procedure and pass ureteric stents. There may be illuminated ones available

4 If the ureter is crushed, transfixed with a suture or divided consult a urologist

5 If in doubt confirm with a cystoscopy and passage of ureteric catheters

---

Bowel injuries

Most injuries are in the form of stitch penetration to the ano-rectum or inadvertent opening into the rectum (proctotomy). The vast majority are extraperitoneal and with appropriate treatment will heal without fistula formation.

ACTION PLAN

1 Suspect and recognize. Get senior help (?surgical if large defect)

2 Lavage (e.g. normal saline: Betadine), good retraction and light

3 Repair in two layers with 2/0 absorbable suture. Ensure haemostasis

4 Attempt to bring a layer of fascial tissue or muscle to interpose between rectal wall and vaginal skin

5 Antibiotic cover. Fluids only 48 hours and low-residue diet 1 week

PROCEDURE SPECIFIC COMPLICATIONS

Sacrospinous ligament fixation

Haemorrhage and neurological complications may occur. Occasionally damage can occur to the bowel.

Primary/delayed haemorrhage

Many large vessels are at risk during this procedure, e.g. pudendal vessels, middle rectal artery and hypogastric venous plexus.

IF PRIMARY HAEMORRHAGE OCCURS

<table>
<tr><td rowspan="3">ACTION PLAN</td><td>1</td><td>Good exposure, light, suction and assistance are essential. A Miyasaki retractor with light source is especially useful in this scenario. The bleeding source can often be identified and ligated or cauterized</td></tr>
<tr><td>2</td><td>General ooze should be treated with tight packing and/or a hydro-static balloon catheter</td></tr>
<tr><td>3</td><td>Delayed haemorrhage may result in the formation of a retroperitoneal haematoma. If this is large and expanding the best recourse is laparotomy (probably with a surgical colleague) and evacuation. Internal iliac ligation may be required</td></tr>
</table>

SUPPLEMENTARY INFORMATION

Self-limiting haematomas should be treated conservatively and the patient commenced on antibiotics. Spontaneous rupture may occur through the vagina which will usually lead to symptomatic improvement and should be managed conservatively. The main risk is of infected haematoma which can be life-threatening and/or result in fistula formation e.g. recto-vaginal.

Neurological complications

Gluteal pain occurs after 3–15% of fixations and is probably secondary to injury of small nerves that run through the ligament.

Mild to moderate pain

<table>
<tr><td rowspan="3">ACTION PLAN</td><td>1</td><td>Reassure the patient that this is common (it should have been discussed prior to surgery) and typically self-limiting usually completely resolving completely by 6 weeks</td></tr>
<tr><td>2</td><td>Ensure adequate analgesia is provided. NSAIDs are the usual first choice</td></tr>
<tr><td>3</td><td>Explain the mechanism of the pain i.e. damage to small nerves in the sacro-spinous ligament and reassure</td></tr>
</table>

Severe or radiating pain

Immediate and severe post-operative gluteal pain radiating down the posterior surface of the leg with or without perineal paraesthesia indicates posterior cutaneous, pudendal or sciatic nerve trauma and requires immediate return to theatre.

ACTION PLAN

1 **Return the patient to theatre**

2 **Remove the suture or sutures**

3 **Resuspension should be performed in a more medial position on the same or opposite side**

Abdominal sacrocolpopexy

A specific and potentially life-threatening complication is trauma to the presacral vessels when attaching the 'graft' to the sacrum. This can be very difficult to control as a result of retraction of the vessels into the periosteum.

ACTION PLAN

1 **Attempt suturing and coagulation**

2 **The insertion of a sterile thumb-tack to compress the bleeding vessel and periosteum may be life-saving**

Abdominal enterocele repairs (e.g. Moschowitz, Halban, uterosacral plication)

The main risk here is of ureteric obstruction secondary to suture entrapment or ureteric kinking. This can be avoided by identification of the ureter and careful suture placement. Occasionally one can make releasing incisions in the peritoneum lateral to the uterosacral ligaments to prevent excessive kinking.

ACTION PLAN

1 Suspect and palpate

2 Carry out a cystoscopy and pass ureteric catheters to make palpation of the ureter easier

3 Remove the suture if it is damaging or acutely kinking the ureter

4 Consider a relieving incision in the peritoneum to release the ureter

FURTHER READING

Walters MD and Karram MM (Eds) (1999) *Urogynecology And Reconstructive Pelvic Surgery,* 2nd edn. Mosby, London.

GYNAECOLOGICAL EMERGENCIES IN OVARIAN CANCER

Susan Houghton and Charles Cox

PRESENTATION

Many patients with ovarian cancer present with vague gastrointestinal symptoms, urinary frequency and/or urgency or a pelvic abdominal mass.

In advanced disease they can present as an emergency with:

- Abdominal pain – due to torsion or infarction of the tumour or due to obstruction of an intra-abdominal viscus.
- Rapid abdominal distension – due to tumour growth or ascites.
- Partial or total bowel obstruction – due to extrinsic pressure on the bowel, infiltration of the mesenteries and/or a direct toxic effect decreasing bowel activity.
- Urinary tract obstruction – due to ureteric obstruction.
- Uterovaginal prolapse – due to the increased intra-abdominal pressure.
- Cardiorespiratory compromise – due to gross ascites or pleural effusion.

ACTION PLAN

1 **Pre-operative investigations**
- FBC.
- U&E's.
- LFTS.
- CXR.
- Pelvic/abdominal USS.
- CT scan pelvis/abdomen – may be useful to delineate tumour.
- CA 125.
- β HCG, α-fetoprotein, CEA – if patients young and germ cell tumour suspected.

2 **Treatment**
- Primary debulking or cytoreductive surgery – the aim is to perform accurate staging of the disease and achieve total macroscopic clearance. Minimal residual disease is achieved if no tumour mass greater than 1 cm^3 is left. It involves:
  1 Staging laparotomy via midline or paramedian incision.
  2 Comprehensive inspection of the entire abdominal contents, including diaphragm and peritoneum.
  3 Sampling of ascites or the taking of peritoneal washings.
  4 Removal of all visible tumour (cytoreduction).
  5 TAH BSO, infracolic omentectomy.
  6 Pelvic and para-aortic lymph node sampling.
  7 Resection of any involved bowel.
  8 Documentation of clinical findings at laparotomy.

Complications are as for laparotomy for gynaecological malignancy.
- Adjuvant chemotherapy – used in patients with advanced disease (stage II–IV). Paclitaxel (Taxol) in combination with a platinum therapy

(cisplatin or carboplatin) should be the standard initial therapy (NICE 2000). Paclitaxel/platinum combination chemotherapy is also recommended in recurrent (or resistant) ovarian cancer if the patient has not previously received this drug combination (NICE 2000).

- Interval debulking surgery (IDS) – a second laparotomy performed during the course of chemotherapy to achieve secondary cytoreduction in patients with bulky residual disease. Complications are as for laparotomy.
- Second-look laparotomy – a laparotomy performed after 6–12 courses of chemotherapy to determine whether the patient with a complete clinical response is surgically and pathologically free of disease. It should now only be performed within clinical trials and complications are as for laparotomy.
- Secondary cytoreductive surgery – patients with persistent or recurrent pelvic and abdominal tumours after primary therapy for ovarian cancer occasionally undergo surgical excision of their disease. Complications are as for laparotomy.

CONSULT OTHER TOPICS

Complications of chemotherapy in gynaecological malignancy (p 194)
Complications of laparotomy for gynaecological malignancy (p 190)

REFERENCES

Guidance on the use of Taxanes for Ovarian Cancer. NICE, May 2000.
Guthrie D, Davy MLJ and Philips PR (1984) Study of 656 patients with early ovarian cancer. *Gynecol. Oncol.* **17**: 363–369.
Janicke F, Holscher M, Kuhn W *et al.* (1992) Radical surgical procedure improves survival time in patients with recurrent ovarian cancer. *Cancer* **70**: 2129–2136.
Van der Berg M, Van Lent M, Buyse M *et al.* (1995) The effect of debulking surgery after induction chemotherapy on the prognosis in advanced epithelial ovarian cancer. *N. Engl. J. Med.* **332**: 629–634.

GYNAECOLOGICAL EMERGENCIES IN CANCER OF THE FALLOPIAN TUBE

PRESENTATION

Primary carcinoma of the fallopian tube is rare. Most tubal malignancies are secondary from the uterus or ovary or arise from malignant disease from the GI tract. Primary adenocarcinoma of the fallopian tube can present with variable, non-specific symptoms:

- Abdominal pain.
- Serosanguinous discharge. } this triad of symptoms is known as *hydrops tubae profluens.*
- Pelvic mass.
- Abnormal vaginal bleeding.
- Unexplained abnormal cervical cytology.
- Urinary or bowel disturbance.

ACTION PLAN

1 **Pre-operative investigations**
- FBC.
- U and E's.
- LFTS.
- CXR.
- Pelvic/abdominal USS.
- CT scan pelvis/abdomen – may be useful to delineate tumour.
- CA 125 – may be elevated in tubal carcinoma.

2 **Treatment**
- Laparotomy – primary debulking surgery is performed as described for ovarian cancer. Staging of the disease is surgical and the tumour is bilateral in 10–20% of cases. Complication are as for laparotomy.
- Adjuvant chemotherapy – cisplatin-based combination chemotherapy has been used in tubal carcinoma with up to an 80% response rate.

CONSULT OTHER TOPICS

Complications of chemotherapy in gynaecological malignancy (p 194)
Complications of laparotomy for gynaecological malignancy (p 190)
Gynaecological emergencies in ovarian cancer (p 169)

GYNAECOLOGICAL EMERGENCIES IN UTERINE CANCER

ENDOMETRIAL CARCINOMA

Presentation

Most endometrial carcinomas present with abnormal vaginal bleeding, especially post-menopausal bleeding, which may be profuse, or inter-menstrual bleeding if pre- or peri-menopausal.

Other presenting symptoms include:

- Abdominal pain.
- Pelvic mass – due to enlarged uterus.
- Pyometra – bloody vaginal discharge due to obstruction of the lower uterine cavity which becomes distended with infected secretions.
- Abnormal glandular cytology or endometrial cells on cervical cytology.

1 **Pre-operative investigations**
- FBC.
- U and E's.
- LFTS.
- CXR.
- Pipelle endometrial biopsy sampling.
- TV ultrasound of the pelvis – to measure endometrial thickness and exclude ovarian pathology.
- CT abdomen and pelvis – especially in obese patients.
- Hysteroscopy, dilatation and curettage – to confirm malignant histology and assess uterine size.

2 **Treatment**
- Staging laparotomy through a midline incision
  1 Total abdominal hysterectomy and bilateral salpingo-oophorectomy.
  2 Peritoneal washings.
  3 Pelvic and para-aortic lymph node sampling in high risk women.
    Complications are as for laparotomy for gynaecological malignancy.
- Vaginal hysterectomy – in patients with marked obesity or medical problems placing them at high risk of complications from abdominal surgery. Complications of vaginal hysterectomy include:
  1 Vaginal bleeding – requiring suturing of the vaginal vault.
  2 Intra-abdominal bleeding - bleeding from a pedicle requiring laparotomy.
  3 Infected vault haematoma – often settle with antibiotics, but may require surgical drainage.
- Adjuvant radiotherapy – is given to decrease vaginal vault and pelvic recurrences. It is not required in patients with Grade 1 or 2 tumours confined to the inner third of the myometrium.
  1 Intracavity radiation (brachytherapy) reduces the incidence of vault recurrence without the increased morbidity of teletherapy (external beam irradiation).

2 Extended-field radiation is given to patients at risk of pelvic lymph node metastases, i.e. biopsy-proven para-aortic nodal metastasis, grossly enlarged or multiple positive pelvic nodes, adenexal metastases, outer-third myometrial invasion or Grade 2 or 3 tumours.
- Recurrent endometrial cancer
  1 In isolated vaginal recurrence surgical excision should be considered if wide normal tissue margins can be achieved followed by radiotherapy if not previously irradiated. This may involve pelvic exenteration.
  2 If surgery is not appropriate and no previous radiotherapy has been given, a combination of teletherapy followed by brachytherapy is given.
  3 In patients with more extensive recurrence medroxyprogesterone acetate 160 mg daily is used with up to a 10% complete response rate.
  4 Recurrent disease is also sensitive to palliation with cisplatin and doxorubicin combination chemotherapy but its use is limited by its toxicity.

UTERINE SARCOMAS

Uterine sarcomas are mesodermal tumours and account for 3% of uterine cancers. They are a heterogeneous group of tumours without standardized treatment protocols.

Presentation

Leiomyosarcomas usually arise *de novo* from uterine smooth muscle but can develop in a pre-exisiting fibroid, which may present with rapid enlargement. Patients may also present with pain, abnormal uterine bleeding or a pelvic abdominal mass. Endometrial stromal sarcomas account for 15–20% of uterine sarcomas and are pre-menopausal in more than 50% of patients. Mixed mesodermal tumours usually occur in postmenopausal women and the tumour often protrudes through the cervical os like a polyp.

Treatment

- Surgical excision – usually Total Abdominal Hysterectomy and Bilateral Salphingo Oophorectomy (TAH and BSO), but young women with a leiomyosarcoma may have ovarian preservation.
- Adjuvant radiotherapy – improves tumour control in the pelvis and may improve survival in surgical Stage I or II disease. Complete response rates of up to 8% have been achieved with combination doxorubicin, cisplatin and ifosfamide.

CONSULT OTHER TOPICS

Complications of chemotherapy in gynaecological malignancy (p 194)
Complications of laparotomy for gynaecological malignancy (p 190)
Complications of radiotherapy in gynaecological malignancy (p 196)

REFERENCE

Knocke TH, Kucera H, Dotfler D, Pokrajac B and Potter R (1998) Results of post-operative radiotherapy in the treatment of sarcoma of the corpus uteri. *Cancer* **83**: 1972–1979.

GYNAECOLOGICAL EMERGENCIES IN CERVICAL CANCER

PRESENTATION

Cervical carcinoma often presents early with:

- Abnormal vaginal bleeding – post-coital, inter-menstrual or post-menopausal. Bleeding may be haemorrhagic requiring:
  1 Resuscitation.
  2 Vaginal packing.
  3 Emergency surgery.
  4 Pelvic irradiation.
- Vaginal discharge – often bloodstained.
- Abnormal cervical cytology – with detection on subsequent colposcopy.

Late disease presents with:

- Malodorous vaginal discharge – infection of tumour bulk with anaerobes.
- Pelvic pain – due to infiltration of the pelvic side walls.
- Referred leg pain – due to invasion of the lumbrosacral plexus.
- Bowel or bladder disturbance – constipation, tenesmus, rectal bleeding, urinary frequency, haematuria or vaginal passage of urine or faeces if a fistula is present.
- Pelvic mass – in advanced disease.

A cervical tumour mass is usually visible either macroscopically or colposcopically.

1 **Pre-operative investigations**
- FBC.
- U and E's.
- LFTS.
- CXR.
- Intravenous pyelogram (IVP) – required for staging of tumour.
- CT scan pelvis/abdomen – assesses liver, urinary tract and bony structures and identifies lymphadenopathy.
- MRI pelvis/abdomen – determines tumour size, degree of stromal penetration, vaginal and parametrial extension and lymph node status. Safe in pregnancy.
- Colposcopy – to assess tumour size, site and vaginal involvement.
- Clinical staging of tumour – staging is clinical and should be performed by an experienced clinician. It includes:
  1 EUA – including a combined recto-vaginal examination to assess the parametrium.
  2 Cervical biopsy – to confirm malignant diagnosis, histologic type, depth of invasion and site of tumour.
  3 Cystoscopy – urine for cytology with biopsy if suspected bladder involvement.
  4 Sigmoidoscopy – with rectal biopsy if suspected rectal involvement.
  5 CXR.
  6 IVP.

2 **Treatment. Cervical tumours more advanced than Stage Ia and all adenocarcinomas should be managed by specialist gynaecological oncologists in approved cancer centres (NHS Executive 1999). Multidisciplinary teams should decide individualized treatment**

- Early stage squamous carcinoma of the cervix (up to Stage Ib1) is treated equally effectively by either surgery or radiotherapy. Surgery is more appropriate for early stage disease, especially in younger women.
- Stage Ib2 disease is probably best treated with pre-operative chemoradiation (consisting of external beam and intracavity caesium with weekly cisplatin) and adjuvant hysterectomy.
- Small volume Stage IIa disease may be amenable to radical surgery.
- Lymph node dissection (LND) is undertaken in Stage Ia2 and more advanced disease.
- Five large Phase III studies in the USA have shown overall survival advantages when cisplatin chemoradiation is used in the treatment of locally advanced (stage IIb–IV) or high-risk cervical cancer as opposed to radiotherapy or surgery alone. It is not yet clear which cytotoxics are the best to combine with radiotherapy.
- Chemoradiation with cisplatin is now considered the standard treatment for inoperable Stage Ib, IIa and IIb disease. It may also be superior to radiation alone in the treatment of Stage IIIb and IVa cancers without para-aortic lymph node involvement.

3 **Summary of surgical treatment of cervical cancer**
- Stage Ia1:
  1 LLETZ.
  2 Knife cone biopsy.
  3 Simple hysterectomy – complications as for laparotomy.
- Stage Ia2:
  1 Knife cone biopsy.
  2 Wertheim's hysterectomy and LND.
  3 Radical trachelectomy – vaginal procedure with excision of cervix, upper vagina and parametrium (uterine body is left in-situ). Immediate complications are infection and bleeding.
- Stage Ib1:
  1 Wertheim's hysterectomy and LND.
- Stage Ib2:
  1 Pre-operative chemoradiation and adjuvant hysterectomy.
- Stage Iia:
  1 Schauta radical vaginal hysterectomy and LND – involves taking a vaginal cuff, often with enlargement of the vaginal orifice with a Schuchardt's incision (like a large mediolateral episiotomy). Decreased operative mortality c.f. Wertheim's, complications as that for vaginal hysterectomy with increased risk of ureteric damage.
- Recurrent cervical cancer: Pelvic recurrence after surgery is treated with radiotherapy. In pelvic recurrence after radiotherapy pelvic exenteration is considered in those fit for such major surgery:
  1 Anterior exenteration involves removal of the bladder, uterus and anterior vagina with construction of a urinary conduit.
  2 Posterior exenteration involves removal of the rectum, uterus and posterior vagina with construction of a stoma.
  3 Total exenteration involves removal of the bladder, urethra, uterus, vagina and rectum with construction of a conduit and stoma.

CONSULT OTHER TOPICS

Complications of chemotherapy in gynaecological malignancy (p 194)
Complications of exenterative surgery for gynaecological malignancy (p 178)
Complications of laparotomy for gynaecological malignancy (p 190)
Complications of large loop excision of the transformation zone (p 192)
Complications of radiotherapy in gynaecological malignancy (p 196)
Complications of Wertheim's hysterectomy and lymph node dissection for cervical cancer (p 177)

REFERENCES

Keys HM, Bundy BN, Stehman FB *et al*. (1999) Cisplatin, radiation and adjuvant hysterectomy compared with radiation and adjuvant hysterectomy for bulky Stage Ib cervical carcinoma. *N. Engl. J. Med.* **340(15):** 1154–1161.

Morris M, Eifel PJ, Lu J *et al*. (1999) Pelvic radiation with concurrent chemotherapy compared with pelvic and para-aortic radiation for high-risk cervical cancer. *N. Engl. J. Med.* **340(15):** 1137–1143.

NHS Executive (1999) Guidance On Commissioning Cancer Services. Improving Outcomes in Gynaecological Cancers. The Manual. NHS Executive, 1999.

Peters WA III, Liu PY, Barrett RJ *et al*. (2000) Cisplatin and 5-FU plus radiation therapy are superior to radiation therapy as an adjunctive in high-risk early-stage carcinoma of the cervix after radical hysterectomy and pelvic lymphadenectomy: report of a phase III intergroup study. *J. Clin. Oncol.* **18:** 450.

Rose PG, Bundy BN, Watkins EB *et al*. (1999) Concurrent cisplatin-based radiotherapy for locally advanced cervical cancer. *N. Engl. J. Med.* **(15):** 1144–1153.

Whitney CW, Sause W, Bundy BN *et al*. (1999) Randomized comparison of fluorouracil plus cisplatin versus hydroxyurea as an adjunct to radiation therapy in stage IIB–IVA carcinoma of the cervix with negative para-aortic nodes: a Gynecologic Oncology Group and Southwest Oncology Group study. *J. Clin. Oncol.* **17(5):** 1339–1348.

COMPLICATIONS OF WERTHEIM'S HYSTERECTOMY AND LYMPH NODE DISSECTION FOR CERVICAL CANCER

1 **Complications as for laparotomy for gynaecological malignancy**

2 **Haemorrhage can occur at the ureteric tunnel, paracolpos and vaginal edge, external iliac artery and vein, obturator fossa, bifurcation of common iliac artery and vein and from para-aortic lymph nodes**
- Use of regional anaesthesia reduces small vessel oozing.
- Direct pressure. } can arrest
- Ligation of vessels. } bleeding

3 **Ureteric dysfunction due to damage to the ureteric nerve or blood supply, oedema of the ureteric wall or periureteric infection in the retroperitoneal space**

4 **Ureteric stricture and uretero-vaginal fistulae develop late and may require surgery**

5 **Bladder dysfunction due to:**
- Damage to sympathetic nerves in the utero-sacral and cardinal ligaments resulting in bladder hypertonicity due to the parasympathetic nerves.
- Oedema of bladder neck and muscle.
- Hypotonicity as a result of over distension of a hypertonic bladder. (Catherization for 6–8 days post-operatively is recommended.) Bifurcation of common iliac artery and vein para-aortic lymph nodes.

6 **Urinary tract infection**

7 **Vesico-vaginal fistulae**

8 **Pelvic lymphocysts of the pelvic brim or pelvic sidewall can cause pain, obstruction or become infected**
- Surgical drainage may be required.

9 **Peripheral leg lymphoedema may develop late**
- Requires specialized massage.

10 **Nerve damage to the obturator, genito-femoral, femoral, perineal or sciatic nerves**

11 **Sexual dysfunction – this is increased if patient receives adjuvant radiotherapy**

CONSULT OTHER TOPICS

Complications of laparotomy for gynaecological malignancy (p 190)
Gynaecological emergencies in cervical cancer (p 174)

COMPLICATIONS OF EXENTERATIVE SURGERY FOR GYNAECOLOGICAL MALIGNANCY

INTRA-OPERATIVE COMPLICATIONS

1 Haemorrhage – increased if previous radiotherapy to pelvis

2 Fluid loss – must be carefully monitored and replaced by the anaesthetist

3 Bowel trauma – increased risk if previous radiotherapy

POST-OPERATIVE COMPLICATIONS

1 Secondary haemorrhage – especially from the ligated internal iliac arteries and pelvic floor musculature
- Direct pressure.
- Ligation of vessels.
- Intra-abdominal packing.

2 Thromboembolic disease
- Adequate hydration, TED stockings, thromboprophylaxis and early mobilization.

3 Pelvic and wound infection
- Pre-operative bowel preparation with picolax is essential.
- Prophylactic antibiotics should be continued post-operatively.

4 Empty pelvis syndrome includes malaise, pyrexia with rigors and perineal sinus discharge

5 Biochemical disturbance – acid–base disturbance, hyperkalaemia, jaundice, raised LFTs, hypoproteinaemia, low magnesium and zinc levels
- Careful monitoring and adequate correction of metabolic disturbance is essential.
- Parenteral nutrition may be required.

6 Intestinal obstruction and fistulae are usually intestino-perineal, especially ileo-perineal due to loops of ileum falling into the pelvis and compromising their blood supply. The risk of ileo-perineal fistulae is increased if an ileal conduit is constructed

7 **Urological complications**
- Early complications include urine spillage at surgery, urine leakage at the uretero-conduit junction, conduit infarction, conduit torsion, blockage of the conduit stents and urinary tract infection.
- Late complications include urinary tract infection, fistula, ureteric stricture or stenosis, renal and conduit stones, metabolic disturbance and stoma tumour recurrence.

8 **Psychosexual problems**
- Pre-operative counseling is of paramount importance.

CONSULT OTHER TOPICS

Complications of laparotomy for gynaecological malignancy (p 190)
Gynaecological emergencies in cervical cancer (p 174)

GYNAECOLOGICAL EMERGENCIES IN VAGINAL CANCER

PRESENTATION

Vaginal cancer accounts for 1–2% of gynaecological malignancies. Most vaginal carcinomas are secondary, especially of the cervix, endometrium, colon or rectum. Up to 30% of primary vaginal cancers occur in patients with a history of pre-invasive or invasive cervical cancer. Vaginal intraepithelial neoplasia (VAIN) is a precursor, but its malignant potential is unknown. Nine percent of primary vaginal malignancies are adenocarcinomas and may be related to exposure to diethylstilbestrol *in utero*.

Patients present with:

- Vaginal bleeding or discharge.
- Dysuria.
- Urinary frequency.
- Pelvic pain.
- Pelvic mass.
- Tenesmus.

ACTION PLAN

Careful inspection of the vaginal walls whilst withdrawing the bivalve speculum is required to identify the tumour, which is commonly present in the upper one third of the vagina.

1 **Pre-operative investigations**
- FBC.
- U&E's.
- LFTS.
- CXR.
- IVP.
- CT scan or MRI of pelvis/abdomen.
- Clinical staging of the tumour involves:
  1 EUA with combined rectovaginal examination.
  2 Full thickness biopsy.
  3 Cystoscopy.
  4 Sigmoidoscopy.

2 **Treatment. There is no consensus as to the correct management of primary vaginal cancer. Treatment is individualized and for most patients maintenance of a functional vagina is important**
- Radiotherapy – most patients are treated with radiotherapy consisting of a combination of teletherapy (external beam radiotherapy) and brachytherapy (intracavity or interstitial therapy). The mid-tumour dose should be at least 75 Gy. Vaginal necrosis may occur and vaginal stenosis occurs in between 13% and 48%. If the lower third of the vagina is involved, the inguinal nodes should be treated or dissected.
- Surgery – has a limited role in the management of patients with vaginal cancer. It is considered in:

1 Stage I disease involving the upper posterior vagina – involves radical hysterectomy, partial vaginectomy and bilateral pelvic lymphadecectomy.

2 Small, low, mobile Stage I tumours – involves vulvectomy with inguinal lymphadenectomy.

3 Young patients who require radiotherapy – pre-treatment laparotomy allows ovarian transposition, surgical staging and resection of enlarged lymph nodes.

4 Stage IVa disease, particularly if recto-vaginal or vesico-vaginal fistula present – pelvic exenteration may be appropriate.

5 Patients with a central recurrence after radiotherapy – often involves pelvic exenteration.

- Chemotherapy – combined chemoradiation has been used as first-line treatment for advanced disease and palliative chemotherapy for recurrent disease. Cisplatin, 5-fluorouracil and mitomycin-C have been used.

CONSULT OTHER TOPICS

REFERENCES

Dancuart F, Delclos L, Taylor WJ and Silva EG (1988) Primary squamous cell carcinoma of the vagina treated by radiotherapy: a failure analysis – The MD Anderson experience 1955–1982. *Int. J. Radiat. Oncol. Biol. Phys.* **14:** 745–749.

Kirkbride P, Fyles A, Rawlings GA *et al.* (1995) Carcinoma of the vagina – experience at the Princess Margaret Hospital (1974–1989). *Gynecol. Oncol.* **56:** 435–443.

Nanavati PJ, Fanning J, Hilgers RD, Hallstrom, J and Crawford D (1993) High-dose-rate brachytherapy in primary stage I and II vaginal cancer. *Gynecol. Oncol.* **51:** 67–71.

COMPLICATIONS OF VAGINECTOMY FOR VAGINAL CANCER

1 **Intra-operative haemorrhage**
- Direct pressure.
- Ligation of bleeding vessels.
- Intra-abdominal packing.
- Internal iliac artery ligation.

2 **Trauma to bladder or rectum**
- Primary repair.
- Resection and anastomosis.
- Defunctioning colostomy.
- Formation of ileal conduit.

3 **Fixity of bladder base – scarring of bladder base can fix the urethra causing retention or incontinence**

4 **Loss of all or part of the vagina**

5 **Shortening and scarring of the vagina**
- Skin grafting may be required.

6 **Fistulae formation**
- Surgery may be required.

CONSULT OTHER TOPICS

Complications of exenterative surgery for gynaecological malignancy (p 178)
Gynaecological emergencies in vaginal cancer (p 180)

GYNAECOLOGICAL EMERGENCIES IN VULVAL CANCER

PRESENTATION

Carcinoma of the vulva comprises 3–5% of all gynaecological malignancies. Ninety percent are squamous carcinomas. Most vulval cancers present in elderly women and are associated with maturation disorders including lichen sclerosus and Paget's disease. Vulval cancer in younger women is associated with HPV infection, smoking and VIN.

Women with vulval cancer may be asymptomatic or can present with:
1. Puritus – often present for many years.
2. A vulval lump or mass.
3. A vulval ulcer.
4. Vulval bleeding or discharge.
5. Dysuria.
6. Metastatic groin mass.

ACTION PLAN

1 Pre-operative investigations
- FBC.
- U&E's.
- LFTs.
- CXR.
- Pelvic USS.
- Cervical smear.
- Colposcopy of cervix and vagina – squamous vulval carcinoma is associated with other squamous lesions of the lower genital tract.
- Radiological assessment of the groins – to assess inguinal lymphadenopathy.
- Wedge or excision biopsy – to include the transitional area between normal tissue and tumour and underlying dermis and connective tissue to determine stromal invasion.
- Biopsy or fine-needle aspiration of enlarged inguinal lymph nodes.

2 Treatment
- Surgery – staging of vulval cancer is surgical and management should be undertaken in Gynaecological Cancer Centres by multidisciplinary teams with specialist nursing expertise (RCOG, 1999).
  1 Treatment is individualized depending upon the site, size and stage of the tumour, the histologic type, groin node status and excision margins.
  2 Wide radical local excision should include a margin of at least 1 cm of normal tissue.
  3 Groin lymph node dissection should include superficial and deep inguino-femoral dissection.

3 Summary of surgical management of vulval cancer (early disease)
- Stage Ia (small lesions with < 1 mm invasion).
  1 Wide local excision.
- Lateralized Stage I/II squamous lesions (medial edge of tumour is at least 2 cm lateral to the midline of the vulva).

1 Wide local excision and ipsilateral groin LND (if groin nodes positive will require contra-lateral groin LND or irradiation).
- Centrally located tumours where excision is possible without sphincter compromise.
  1 Wide local excision and bilateral groin LND (large and multifocal tumours may require triple incision radical vulvectomy).

4 **Summary of surgical management of vulval cancer (advanced disease)**
- Extensive vulval involvement.
  1 Primary radiotherapy to vulva with bilateral groin LND (may require surgical excision and vulval reconstruction).
- Clinically advanced nodes.
  2 Surgical excision.
  3 Chemoradiation.
- Metastatic disease.
  1 Palliation (may require appropriate management of primary tumour).
- Radiotherapy and chemotherapy – radiotherapy, with or without concurrent chemotherapy (5 fluorouracil), is indicated:
  1 Before surgery in patients with advanced disease who would otherwise require pelvic exenteration.
  2 Post-operatively as adjuvant treatment to the inguinal and deep pelvic lymph nodes in patients with macroscopic involvement of one node, 2 or more histologically proven positive nodes or extracapsular spread.
  3 As treatment of local vulval and groin recurrences.
- Recurrent vulval carcinoma.
  1 In local recurrence radiotherapy should be used if excision would impair sphincter function.
  2 Excision should be considered if maximum dose radiotherapy has already been given.
  3 In histologically confirmed groin recurrence radiotherapy should be given to patients not previously irradiated.
  4 Resection should be considered if the response to radiotherapy is partial or as palliation in patients previously irradiated.

CONSULT OTHER TOPICS

Complications of chemotherapy in gynaecological malignancy (p 194)
Complications of exenterative surgery for gynaecological malignancy (p 178)
Complications of radiotherapy in gynaecological malignancy (p 196)
Complications of the surgical management of vulval cancer (p 185)

REFERENCES

Byfield JE, Calabro-Jones P, Klisak I and Kulhanian F (1982) Pharmacologic requirements for obtaining sensitization of human tumour cells in vitro to combined 5 fluorouracil or ftorafur and X-rays. *Int. J. Radiat. Oncol. Biol. Phys.* **8:** 1923–1932.
Homesley HD, Bundy BN, Sedlis A and Adcock L (1986) Radiation therapy versus node resection for carcinoma of the vulva with positive groin nodes. *Obstet. Gynecol.* **68:** 733–740.
RCOG Clinical Recommendations for the Management of Vulval Cancer. July 1999.
Thomas G, Dembo A, DePetrillo A *et al*. (1989) Concurrent radiation and chemotherapy in vulvar carcinoma. *Gynecol. Oncol.* **34:** 263–267.

COMPLICATIONS OF THE SURGICAL MANAGEMENT OF VULVAL CANCER

INTRA-OPERATIVE COMPLICATIONS

ACTION PLAN

1 **Haemorrhage**
- Direct pressure.
- Ligation of bleeding vessels.

EARLY COMPLICATIONS

ACTION PLAN

1 **Wound breakdown**
- Bed rest is advised for 3–5 days to foster healing.

2 **Wound infection and necrosis**
- Use prophylactic antibiotics.
- Infected wounds should be debrided, irrigated and appropriately dressed.

3 **DVT and PE**
- Adequate hydration, TED stockings, thromboprophylaxis and early mobilization.

4 **MI – up to 2% post-operatively mortality due to MI or PE**
- Observe carefully for symptoms and signs of MI.
- Perform ECG.
- If MI suspected:
  1 CHECK AIRWAY, BREATHING AND CIRCULATION.
  2 Give oxygen via a face mask at 15 l/min.
  3 Give 5 mg diamorphine slowly iv over 5 minutes.
  4 Give 10 mg metoclopramide iv.
  5 Give 150 mg aspirin (chewed or dispersed in water).
  6 Refer to Medics for appropriate treatment and discuss use of thrombolytic drugs e.g. streptokinase.

5 **Secondary haemorrhage – significant ooze can occur from the groin wounds**
- Groin drains should be left *in-situ* post-operatively.

6 **Pressure sores**
- Should be managed by appropriately trained staff.

7 **Femoro-inguinal lymphocyst – occur in up to 30%**
- If infected, they should be incised and broad-spectrum antibiotics prescribed.

8 **Urinary tract infections**
- A Foley catheter is left *in-situ* until the patient is ambulatory.

LATE COMPLICATIONS

1 **Chronic leg lymphoedema**
- Use prophylactic compression stockings post-operatively.
- Elevation of the limbs at rest.
- Exercise of limbs.
- Use of compression stockings.
- Massage by specialist nurses or physiotherapists.

2 **Recurrent lymphangitis – common in patients with chronic lymphoedema, who may become severely shocked and toxic**
- Treat with broad-spectrum antibiotics and intravenous rehydration.

3 **Urinary dysfunction – stress incontinence and difficulties in directing the urinary stream may occur**

4 **Genital prolapse – probably due to loss of the perineal supporting tissues and/or nerve damage to the muscles around the introitus**
- May require corrective surgery.

5 **Introital stenosis**
- May require a vertical relaxing incision.

6 **Faecal incontinence – may occur if the anal sphincter was damaged at initial surgery**

7 **Recto-vaginal or recto-perineal fistulas**
- May require surgery.

8 **Femoral hernia**
- May require surgical repair.

9 **Femoral nerve damage – anterior thigh paraesthesia and pain may develop due to transection of branches of the femoral nerve at groin lymph node dissection**

10 **Psychological and psychosexual dysfunction – altered body image may vary greatly**
- All women need support and counseling to cope with surgery for vulval cancer.

CONSULT OTHER TOPIC

Gynaecological emergencies in vulval cancer (p 183)

EMERGENCIES IN PAEDIATRIC GYNAECOLOGICAL ONCOLOGY

Malignant tumours are rare in childhood and adolescence.

OVARY

- Ovarian tumours are the most common genital tract tumours in girls.
- Less than 1% of all tumours in girls under 16 years of age are ovarian.
- About 30% of childhood ovarian tumours are benign teratomas.
- The most common malignant ovarian tumours in childhood are germ-cell carcinomas, i.e. dysgerminoma, endodermal sinus tumour or malignant teratomas.
- More rare tumours are embryonal carcinoma, primary ovarian choriocarcinoma and mixed germ-cell tumour.

Presentation

Ovarian tumours in childhood often present with:

- Abdominal pain.
- Abdominal mass.
- Urinary frequency.
- Rectal discomfort.
- Anorexia.

Treatment involves:

- Surgical excision by unilateral oophorectomy with pelvic and para-aortic lymph node excision when appropriate.
- Adjuvant post-operative chemotherapy may be indicated.

UTERUS

Uterine tumours are extremely rare in childhood and adolescence.

CERVIX

- The most common tumour of the cervix and vagina in girls under 16 years of age is sarcoma botryoides.
- Ninety percent of girls with sarcoma botryoides present before the age of 5 years.
- Sarcoma botryoides usually arises from the vagina in young girls and the cervix and upper vagina in older girls or adolescents.

Presentation

Eighty percent of girls present with either:

- Abnormal vaginal bleeding.
- Bloody vaginal discharge.
- A vaginal or abdominal mass, which is often grape-like in appearance.

1 **Diagnosis is made by:**
- EUA, including protoscopy and cystoscopy.
- Biopsy.

2 **Treatment**
- Multimodality treatment combining chemotherapy, radiotherapy and less radical surgery has enabled preservation of reproductive function in early stage disease.
- Primary chemotherapy involves triple therapy with vincristine, actinomycin D and cyclophosphamide.

VAGINA

- Clear-cell adenocarcinoma of the vagina is related to vaginal adenosis and exposure to diethylstilboestrol (DES) *in utero*.
- The tumour is usually situated in the upper anterior third of the vagina.

Presentation

- Asymptomatic.
- Vaginal discharge.
- Post-coital bleeding.

ACTION PLAN

1 **Diagnosis is made by**
- Examination Under Anaesthesia (EUA).
- Biopsy.

2 **Treatment**
- Early disease can be treated by wide local excision, lymphadenectomy and adjuvant radiotherapy.
- Advanced disease requires radical surgery and adjuvant radiotherapy.

VULVA

Vulval tumours are extremely rare in childhood and adolescence. These include squamous cell carcinoma, malignant melanomas and sarcoma botryoides.

CONSULT OTHER TOPICS

Complications of chemotherapy in gynaecological malignancy (p 194)
Complications of radiotherapy in gynaecological malignancy (p 196)
Gynaecological emergencies in cancer of the fallopian tube (p 171)
Gynaecological emergencies in cervical cancer (p 174)
Gynaecological emergencies in ovarian cancer (p 169)

REFERENCES

Copeland, LJ, Gershenson, DM, Sau PB *et al.* (1985) Sarcoma botryoides of the female genital tract. *Obstet. Gynecol.* **66:** 262–266.

Hilgers RD, Malkasian GD and Saule EH (1972) Embryonal rhabdomyosarcoma (botryoid type) of the vagina. A clinicopathologic review. *Am. J. Obstet. Gynecol.* **107:** 484–502.

COMPLICATIONS OF LAPAROTOMY FOR GYNAECOLOGICAL MALIGNANCY

Complications of laparotomy for gynaecological malignancy are the same irrespective of primary tumour type.

INTRA-OPERATIVE COMPLICATIONS

1 **Haemorrhage – especially from the infundibulopelvic ligaments or the bed of an incompletely resected pelvic tumour**
   - Direct pressure may arrest bleeding.
   - Use of a haemostatic substance e.g. Surgicell.
   - Internal iliac artery ligation.

2 **Bowel damage – due to direct tumour involvement or adhesion formation**
   - Primary repair of damaged bowel wall.
   - Bowel resection and primary anastomosis.
   - Defunctioning or permanent ileostomy / colostomy.

3 **Ureteric or bladder damage – due to close proximity to tumour or metastases**
   - Primary repair of bladder injury.
   - Primary repair of ureteric injury.
   - Ureteric re-implantation.
   - Uretero-ureterostomy.
   - Formation of ileal conduit.

4 **Damage to large blood vessels – compression or infiltration of external iliac arteries and veins**
   - Direct pressure.
   - Ligation of vessels.

5 **Direct trauma to other intra-abdominal organs – on resection of metastases or due to retraction**
   - Primary repair.
   - Resection of damaged tissue or organ.

POST-OPERATIVE COMPLICATIONS

ACTION PLAN

1 **Ileus**
- Intra-operative NGT insertion.

2 **Wound dehiscence or incisional hernia**
- Mass closure is advised.

3 **Wound infection**
- Give prophylactic antibiotics.

4 **DVT and PE**
- Adequate hydration, TED stockings, thromboprophylaxis and early mobilization.

CONSULT OTHER TOPICS

Gynaecological emergencies in cancer of the fallopian tube (p 171)
Gynaecological emergencies in cervical cancer (p 174)
Gynaecological emergencies in ovarian cancer (p 169)
Gynaecological emergencies in uterine cancer (p 172)
Gynaecological emergencies in vaginal cancer (p 180)

COMPLICATIONS OF LARGE LOOP EXCISION OF THE TRANSFORMATION ZONE

Large loop excision of the transformation zone (LLETZ) is now the most common treatment for CIN. It has similar complications to cold knife cone biopsy, but they occur less frequently.

INTRA-OPERATIVE COMPLICATIONS

ACTION PLAN

- **Haemorrhage**
1 Anticipate and reduce by intra-cervical infiltration of local anaesthetic (e.g. Citanest, containing 3% prilocaine HCl and 0.03% octapressin).
2 Ball diathermy fulguration should arrest bleeding.
3 Suturing of the cervix with a figure of eight haemostatic suture to a bleeding point.
4 Pack the vagina with large packs and admit for bed rest overnight.
5 Perform an EUA with suturing of cervix if bleeding does not settle.

- **Pain**
1 Usually minimal but may require simple analgesia.
2 Reduced with intra-cervical infiltration of local anaesthetic.

- **Vasovagal attack or fainting**
1 Stop procedure if she feels faint before LLETZ performed.
2 Increase cerebral blood flow by simple measures, e.g. raise foot of couch/bed, put patient's head between her knees.
3 Observe carefully on ward prior to discharge.

POST-OPERATIVE COMPLICATIONS

ACTION PLAN

- **Secondary haemorrhage – excessive bleeding within 3 weeks of treatment, occurs in 4%**
1 If bleeding point identified apply Monsels paste or cauterize with silver nitrate or ball diathermy fulguration.
2 Often related to infection and usually settles with broad spectrum antibiotics.
3 May require bed rest +/– vaginal packing and observation overnight.
4 If bleeding does not settle will require EUA and cervical suturing if bleeding point identified.

- **Vaginal discharge – average duration is 2 weeks, may last up to 6 weeks. If infection suspected take swabs and treat with broad-spectrum antibiotics**

- **Cervical stenosis – occurs in < 2%**
1 If symptomatic will require cervical dilatation.
2 Can usually be performed under local anaesthetic.

CONSULT OTHER TOPIC

Gynaecological emergencies in cervical cancer (p 174)

REFERENCES

Luesley DM, Cullimore, J, Redman CWE *et al.* (1990) Loop diathermy excision of the cervical transformation zone in patients with abnormal cervical smears. *BMJ* **300:** 1690–1693.

Prendiville W, Cullimore J and Norman S (1989) Large loop excision of the transformation zone (LLETZ): a new method of management for women with cervical intraepithelial neoplasia. *Br. J. Obstet. Gynecol.* **96:** 1054–1060.

COMPLICATIONS OF CHEMOTHERAPY IN GYNAECOLOGICAL MALIGNANCY

1 **Haematological – myelosuppression, common with carboplatin, can cause:**
   - Granulocytopenia – predisposing to sepsis. Use prophylatic, broad-spectrum antibiotics in febrile granulocytopenic patients.
   - Thrombocytopenia - with a risk of spontaneous haemorrhage.
   - Anaemia – usually presents after several courses of chemotherapy.

2 **Gastrointestinal**
   - Nausea and vomiting – common side effects.
     1 Use 5-HT$_3$ antagonists.
   - Mucositis – mouth and pharyngeal ulceration, oesophagitis causing dysphagia, bowel ulceration resulting in diarrhoea or necrotizing enterocolitis (NEC) in severe cases with granulocytopenia.
     1 iv hydration with electrolyte replacement.
     2 Antimotility drugs e.g. codeine phosphate.
     3 Vancomycin in NEC.

3 **Genitourinary**
   - Acute renal failure – cisplatin particularly causes dose-related renal tubular toxicity.
     1 Use pre- and post-treatment iv hydration.
   - Haemorrhagic cystitis – due to the irritant effect on the bladder mucosa of acrolein, the toxic metabolite of cyclophosphamide.
     1 Hydration, diuresis and mesna (sodium mercaptoethane sulfonate) help prevent this.
   - Hepatotoxicity – elevation of liver enzymes may occur.
   - Neurotoxicity – many cytotoxics cause some central or peripheral neurotoxicity.
     Cisplatin – produces ototoxicity, peripheral neuropathy, and, rarely, retrobulbar neuritis and blindness.
     Paclitaxel – associated with peripheral sensory neuropathy. Neurotoxicity increased with combination cisplatin therapy.

4 **Immunosuppression – suppression of cellular and humoral immunity predispose to opportunistic infection**

5 **Hypersensitivity reactions – associated with carboplatin, paclitaxel and anaphylaxis with cisplatin**

6 **Alopecia – common with paclitaxel. Usually reversible but associated with significant psychological morbidity**

7 **Gonadal dysfunction**
   - Infertility – many cytotoxics cause infertility. Successful pregnancies have been achieved after cisplatin-based chemotherapy.
   - Teratogenicity – all cytotoxics carry the risk of teratogenicity.

8 **Second malignancies – cisplatin is associated with the development of acute leukaemia**

CONSULT OTHER TOPICS

Complications of Chemotherapy

COMPLICATIONS OF RADIOTHERAPY IN GYNAECOLOGICAL MALIGNANCY

The complications of radiotherapy are dose-dependent and may present either acutely or late, occurring up to many years after treatment.

ACUTE COMPLICATIONS

- Erythema or desquamation of the skin.
- Diarrhoea.
- Bladder irritability – frequency and dysuria.
- Bone marrow suppression – anaemia, thrombocytopenia, neutropenia.

LATE COMPLCATIONS

- Small bowel – subacute or acute bowel obstruction, bleeding, perforation, fistulae and malabsorption.
- Large bowel – proctosigmoiditis, recto-vaginal fistula and recto-sigmoid obstruction, stricture, perforation or fistulous communication with other intra-abdominal organs.
- Bladder – contracture with reduced capacity, heamorrhagic cystitis, vesico-vaginal fistula, ureteric obstruction and hydronephrosis.
- Ovarian failure.
- Vaginal atrophy and stenosis.

CONSULT OTHER TOPICS

Gynaecological emergencies in cervical cancer (p 174)
Gynaecological emergencies in uterine cancer (p 172)
Gynaecological emergencies in vaginal cancer (p 180)
Gynaecological emergencies in vulval cancer (p 183)

Complications of Radiotherapy

HAEMORRHAGE CONTROL

Charles Cox

'All bleeding comes to an end' but not always in ways that ensure a favourable outcome.

The principles of haemorrhage control are to turn off the tap and to replace circulating blood volume. Bleeding is controlled by direct pressure initially. Haemorrhage control will be considered in the situation of hysterectomy, bleeding from the sacrum and pelvis and in the situation where the bleeding is not obviously coming from the pelvic organs.

A laparotomy for hypovolaemic shock is a part of resuscitation, 'the resuscitative laparotomy'.

A familiar example is a lapararotomy for a ruptured ectopic pregnancy where the priority is to stop the bleeding before getting the blood pressure back to normal. The object of resuscitation prior to surgery is for the patient to be 'talking not walking'.

The control of bleeding at laparotomy and the 'trauma' laparotomy will be discussed.

In the majority of cases the cause of haemorrhage in gynaecology will be a ruptured ectopic pregnancy or a laparotomy for post-operative haemorrhage.

In these cases a low transverse incision or reopening the previous incision will be appropriate.

However, if there is a suggestion of trauma or the diagnosis is uncertain a low midline incision, which can be extended above the umbilicus, should be made.

SUSPECTED RUPTURED ECTOPIC PREGNANCY

ACTION PLAN

1 **Make a low transverse incision if confident of the diagnosis (a preliminary laparoscopy should not be carried out on the haemodynamically unstable patient)**

2 **If a massive haemoperitoneum is present do not attempt to suction all the blood before identifying the source of bleeding**

3 **Grasp the uterus and lift it as far as possible up into the wound and identify the cause of the haemorrhage using finger pressure to control the bleeding before dealing definitively with it**

4 **If bleeding from the tube decide whether to remove the tube (the preferred option) or to attempt some form of conservative surgery. In the majority of cases of massive haemorrhage it is unlikely to be feasible to safely conserve the tube and it is very doubtful if fertility is improved**

5 **If the bleeding is not obviously from the tube carefully examine both ovaries. Occasionally significant haemorrrhage arises from a ruptured ovarian cyst**

POST-OPERATIVE COLLAPSE WITH SUSPECTED REACTIONARY HAEMORRHAGE

ACTION PLAN

1 Open existing incision

2 Suck out blood and use packs to mop out blood

3 Examine vault of vagina

4 Be careful when inserting sutures into the angles of the vagina, the ureter is not far away and should be identified as far as possible. This may be difficult with haematoma and bruising

5 Examine the ovarian pedicles, a slipped ligature is a common cause of post-operative haemorrhage. Associated retro-peritoneal haematoma is common

6 Dissect out the ovarian vessel on the side of a retroperitoneal haematoma which will have retracted retroperitoneally and ligate it

7 If the patient has had an omentectomy bleeding from slipped ligatures may be responsible for haemorrhage from the upper abdomen

THE CONTROL OF MASSIVE INTRA-OPERATIVE OR POST-OPERATIVE BLEEDING

The control of bleeding in the pelvis

The control of presacral bleeding

Venous bleeding in the pelvis is particularly difficult to control as the vein walls are thin and when damaged tend to retract into the deep fascia of the pelvis where they are inaccessible.

ACTION PLAN

1 Massive bleeding may need to be controlled by taking control of the aorta either by direct pressure or by exposing the aorta and clamping it

2 Ensure the presence of an anaesthetist experienced in massive haemorrhage as control of fluid replacement and the prevention and correction of clotting disorders is the key to success. Definitive surgical control of bleeding may need to be deferred until this has been achieved. Bleeding in the meantime is controlled by direct pressure

3 Pack. Initially hot packs and direct pressure, a technique using a bag placed in the pelvis with the neck of the bag being brought out through the vagina has been described for bleeding which cannot be controlled by other means the bag is filled with Wertheim packs with the ends coming through the neck of the bag through the vagina. Traction is applied to the neck of the bag to apply pressure to the pelvic side walls. The Wertheim's packs can then be removed at a

later date one at a time through the vagina followed by the bag. The alternative is to firmly pack the pelvis and to go back a day or so later to remove the packs

4   Stainless steel clips can be applied to bleeding points

5   Oxidized cellular gauze and bone wax can be used to reinforce over-sewing of the bleeding points

6   Ligation of the internal iliac arteries – they should be ligated in continuity and the vessel should not be divided. However in the elderly they may be quite fragile and it may be difficult to pass tapes around the vessels to control them. The blood supply to the pelvis however is rich in anastomotic channels and this technique may not be successful

7   If available a cell saver might be used to enable auto-transfusion of the patient's whole blood

8   Stapling of packs to the sacrum may be tried and sterile drawing pins have been used to control haemorrhage over the sacrum

REFERENCE

Rennie J and Cardozo L (1998). The Seven Surgeons of Kings' a fable by Aesop. *Br. J. Obstet. Gynaecol.* **105:** 1241.

MASSIVE INTRA-ABDOMINAL BLEEDING NOT OBVIOUSLY GYNAECOLOGICAL

ACTION PLAN

1   Suspect – if signs of massive intra-abdominal haemorrhage but no suggestion of an ectopic pregnancy otherwise. However, the denial of the possibility of pregnancy does not rule out ectopic pregnancy!

2   Carry out a lower midline incision

3   Grasp the uterus to lift it out of the pelvis so that the gynaecological organs can be inspected for sources of bleeding

4   If no obvious source of bleeding call a general surgical colleague

5   Extend the abdominal incision above the umbilicus and try to see where blood is coming from, use suction and packing. You may require extensive packing to stop haemorrhage

6   The source of intra-abdominal bleeding is not always obvious and a way to find out is to pack the abdomen sequentially and then remove the packs in reverse order as in a 'trauma' laparotomy. Pack until the bleeding stops or slows

7   Pack the pelvis – lift the omentum, transverse colon and small bowel out of the wound, suck and pack the pelvis

8   Pack the infra-colic compartment. This is divided into right and left i.e. either side of the small bowel mesentery. Move the small bowel to the right and suck and pack to the left then to the right. Bleeding from the mesentery and the bowel should be easily identified but

Haemorrhage Control

the source of retroperitoneal bleeding may be more difficult to identify. Consider rupture of renal artery aneurysms and bleeding from
retroperitoneal organs

9   Pack the right upper quadrant. Pull the transverse colon and omen-
    tum down and move to supra-colic compartment. Suck and pack
    over the right lobe of the liver. Potential causes of bleeding are the
    liver, retrohepatic veins, inferior vena cava, the free edge of the less-
    er omentum, duodenum, pancreas, right adrenal and kidney

10 Pack the left upper quadrant. Suck and pack. The most likely cause
    of bleeding is from a ruptured aneurysm of the splenic artery or from
    the spleen itself. Bleeding could also possibly come from the left lobe
    of the liver, diaphragm, stomach, pancreas, adrenal and kidney

11 Enough packs should be placed in the various compartments until
    bleeding slows and it is possible to see roughly where the bleeding
    is coming from

12 At this stage it will be helpful to allow the anaesthetist time to
    catch up with resuscitation before carrying on to any procedures
    which may cause further heavy bleeding

BLEEDING FROM THE LIVER

Dealing with bleeding from the liver is a highly specialized activity and packing
will be the right option for the non-specialist. It is usually effective as bleeding
from the liver is usually venous and low pressure. However, if bleeding is difficult
to control during the wait for a surgeon Pringle's manoeuvre can be carried out.

This involves placing the left index finger in the foramen of Winslow and pinching the portal structures (portal vein, hepatic artery and common bile duct in the
free edge of the lesser omentum. The foramen is identified by following the gall
bladder and cystic duct medially until it meets the free edge of the lesser omentum.
The foramen is immediately posterior. It is safe to compress these structures for
30–60 minutes.

BLEEDING FROM THE SPLEEN

The decision to remove the spleen should be made by a surgeon as there is a tendency to treat splenic injuries conservatively. If there is severe haemorrhage from
a badly damaged spleen it will need to be mobilized in order to gain control of the
splenic vessels and short gastric arteries. The lieno-renal ligament will need to be
divided with scissors as will the attachments between the spleen and the
diaphragm. When ligating and dividing the splenic vessels great care must be
taken not to injure the tail of the pancreas.

FURTHER READING

Definitive Surgical Trauma Skills Course Manual. Royal College of Surgeons of England,
    2001.

UNSUSPECTED GYNAECOLOGICAL MALIGNANCY

Charles Cox and Susan Houghton

The majority of gynaecological malignancies are managed as elective procedures by clinicians with a special interest. However, it is not uncommon for acute presentations of malignant disease to present to general gynaecologists and general surgeons. The on-call general gynaecologist may be called to the general theatre where a surgeon of variable status may have requested assistance. The most likely scenario is of a complication of ovarian disease. Torsion of a mobile ovarian cyst and intestinal obstruction are the most likely diagnoses. If there has been torsion, haemorrhage, rupture or apparent infection of a cyst or an adnexae then it may not be obvious whether the condition is malignant or not.

SUSPECTED OVARIAN DISEASE FOUND AT LAPAROTOMY BY THE SURGEONS

ACTION PLAN

1 Check what operation the patient has consented to

2 Check the age of the patient and parity

3 Check status of the operating surgeon – if you are both trainees call senior assistance, a gynaecological oncologist if available

4 Carry out or repeat a full laparotomy and document findings fully. See Table 1 FIGO staging of ovarian cancer

5 Ensure peritoneal fluid or peritoneal washings are taken for cytology and for culture if indicated

6 Ask the anaesthetist to take blood for tumour markers – at least a CA125

7 If you are the senior surgeon and malignancy is not clinically obvious do the least possible to relieve symptoms and make certain to make full entries in the notes as to what you have done and why

8 Remember that conditions such as actinomycosis and occasionally endometriosis or pelvic inflammatory disease may mimic malignancy

9 Ensure that adequate biopsies are taken

10 Ensure subsequent referral to oncology team

Table 1. FIGO staging of ovarian cancer

Stage

I   Growth limited to the ovaries

IA   Growth limited to one ovary; no ascites
     No tumour on the external surface; capsule intact

IB   Growth limited to both ovaries; no ascites
     No tumour on the external surfaces; capsule intact

IC   Tumour either stage IA or IB but with tumour on the surface of one or
     both ovaries; or with capsule ruptured; or with ascites present contain-
     ing malignant cells or with positive peritoneal washings

II   Growth involving one or both ovaries with pelvic extension

IIA Extension and/or metastases to the uterus and/or tubes

IIB Extension to other pelvic tissues

IIC Tumour either stage IIA or IIB but with tumour on the surface of one or
     both ovaries; or with capsule(s) ruptured; or with ascites present con-
     taining malignant cells or with positive peritoneal washings

III Tumour involving one or both ovaries with peritoneal implants outside the
     pelvis and/or positive retroperitoneal or inguinal nodes. Superficial liver
     metastases equals Stage III. Tumour is limited to the true pelvis but with
     histologically verified malignant extension to small bowel or omentum

III A tumour grossly limited to the true pelvis with negative nodes but
     with histologically confirmed microscopic seedling of abdominal peri-
     toneal surfaces

IIIB Tumour involving one or both ovaries with histologically confirmed
     implants of abdominal peritoneal surfaces, none exceeding 2 cm in
     diameter. Nodes are negative

IIIC Abdominal implants more than 2 cm in diameter and/or positive
     retroperitoneal or inguinal nodes

IV   Growth involving one or both ovaries with distant metastases. If pleural
     effusion is present there must be positive cytology to allot a case to
     stage IV; parenchymal liver metastases equals stage IV

UNSUSPECTED OVARIAN DISEASE FOUND AT LAPAROTOMY FOR SUSPECTED BENIGN GYNAECOLOGICAL PATHOLOGY

ACTION PLAN

1 Check issues of consent – if a woman over 35 is going to theatre for a laparotomy for a possible ovarian cyst then discussion with regard to removal of the ovaries in case of suspicion of malignancy should have taken place

2 Consult gynaecological oncologist if available

3 Take peritoneal fluid or washings for cytology

4 Check baseline CA125 has been taken

5 Carry out a total abdominal hysterectomy and bilateral salpingo-oophorectomy with large omental biopsy

6 Do not resect bowel or carry out a colostomy except in dire emergency without having consent from the patient

7 Inform the oncology team as soon as possible

INTRACTABLE BLEEDING FROM A CERVICAL TUMOUR

It is unusual to have to take a patient to theatre as an acute emergency to deal with bleeding from a cervical tumour. Packing and embolization should be considered if oncologist not available.

ACTION PLAN

1 **Resuscitate the patient**

2 **Consider embolization, consult radiologist**

3 **If haemorrhage is life threatening do the simplest procedure to control it i.e. total abdominal hysterectomy. The ovaries may be removed if appropriate. Do not attempt a formal Wertheims hysterectomy with lymph node dissection even if technically possible if there has been significant haemorrhage. The haemorrhage may be due to infection**

4 **Refer patient to gynaecological oncologist for further advice and management**

APPENDIX 1

PRE-OPERATIVE INVESTIGATION AND FITNESS FOR ANAESTHESIA

Kate Grady and Barry Miller

Fitness for anaesthesia is a risk–benefit decision, taken by surgeon and anaesthetist. The anaesthetist may decide to anaesthetize a patient with a life-threatening condition which can be treated only by surgery, when he would not anaesthetize such a patient for a non-life-threatening condition or he would delay surgery if not immediately life-threatening and the patient could be rendered fitter over a period of time. Honesty is all important in taking these decisions. The anaesthetist must respect the opinion of the surgeon as to what is urgent and the surgeon should attempt to be accurate in this. The anaesthetist must be accurate about the degree of risk.

METHOD OF ANAESTHESIA

General anaesthesia

General anaesthesia (GA) is described as a triad comprising:

- hypnosis (sleep);
- attenuation of sympathetic reflexes which would otherwise occur in response to painful stimuli;
- muscle relaxation.

Drugs which bring about hypnosis are called induction agents. The common ones are propofol, thiopentone and etomidate. They also contribute to the attenuation of sympathetic reflexes. They are usually given to start anaesthesia as a statutory dose. Propofol is sometimes used as an infusion to maintain anaesthesia throughout the operation. This method is known as total intravenous anaesthesia (TIVA). There are sophisticated pieces of equipment which provide simulated feedback loops which maintain steady state concentration and this method is called target controlled infusion (TCI).

Where TIVA is not used, anaesthesia is continued throughout the operation by the patient breathing or being ventilated with nitrous oxide or air and a volatile agent. The volatile agents are isoflurane, enflurane, sevoflurane and halothane.

The sympathetic response is attenuated by analgesic agents. The ones used mostly intraoperatively are fentanyl, alfentanil and morphine.

A degree of muscle relaxation is acquired during any GA but more profound muscle relaxation by specific drugs (such as atracuriam, vecuronium and rocuronium) may be required to provide adequate surgical conditions e.g. for abdominal hysterectomy. If muscle relaxation is to be provided in this way, the patient will be unable to breathe spontaneously and will require controlled ventilation. This is usually done by a ventilator (or occasionally by hand) through an endotracheal tube.

At laparoscopy, peritoneal insufflation and the consequent rise in intra-abdominal pressure, and the combined Trendeleburg and lithotomy positions compromise spontaneous ventilation. This means controlled ventilation, via an endotracheal tube is necessary. In a slim patient undergoing a short laparoscopy, the anaesthetist may choose to use a laryngeal mask instead of an endotracheal tube.

The patient at risk of regurgitation of gastric fluids must be intubated to avoid aspiration when under anaesthesia and to do this requires muscle relaxation. Aspiration happens in the anaesthetized patient because they have lost the protective airway reflexes. Risk of regurgitation is minimized by an adequate period of starvation but there are some patients in whom it is nevertheless, a risk e.g. inadequately starved, the acute abdomen, pregnancy, hiatus hernia. To minimize the time between loss of laryngeal and pharyngeal reflexes and getting the endotracheal tube into the trachea a short acting muscle relaxant such as suxamethonium is used. This is part of a rapid sequence induction technique in which the patient is pre-oxygenated so there is no need for 'bagging' to oxygenate when the patient becomes paralysed and before the endotracheal tube is in place. Cricoid pressure is used until the endotracheal tube is in place and the cuff is inflated.

Antiemetics are frequently given intra-operatively.

Regional anaesthesia

Regional anaesthesia refers to the injection of local anaesthetic +/– a small dose of opioid drug into either the epidural space (space surrounding dura), or to more directly access spinal nerves and spinal cord opiate receptors, into the cerebrospinal fluid – a spinal (intra-thecal) injection. A spinal requires a much smaller dose of drug, has a more profound therapeutic effect, is of quicker onset and causes greater falls in blood pressure.

PHYSIOLOGICAL EFFECTS OF ANAESTHESIA

Anaesthesia aims to:

- maintain adequate oxygenation;
- maintain adequate blood flow to vital organs, heart, brain, gut, liver, kidney;
- keep the patient asleep;
- provide adequate operating conditions for the surgeon;
- wake the patient up in a comfortable condition.

If there is compromise in any of the organs/systems it is even more important to maintain good oxygenation and flow.

Maintain oxygenation

- This requires a clear airway and adequate ventilation.

Maintain adequate blood flow to vital organs

Oxygen flux equation (oxygenation and flow)

Oxygen flow to any organ depends on cardiac output (CO) (blood flow to organ), haemoglobin (to carry oxygen) and oxygen saturation (saturation of haemoglobin with oxygen).

For this to work, optimization of respiratory system, adequate CO and Hb above 10 g/dl are needed.

Anaesthesia brings about an alteration in respiratory dynamics which compromises ventilation and therefore oxygenation. This is why anaesthetized patients are given at least 30% oxygen in their mixture of inspired gases (compared to the 21% in air). The respiratory mechanics must be such that if controlled ventilation is required it can be carried out adequately and safely. The respiratory system must be robust enough to withstand the effect of the altered dynamics.

Induction agents and volatile agents depress myocardial contractility and cause a fall in vascular resistance and therefore in venous return back to the heart. This can severely affect cardiac output and therefore flow to the vital organs. Controlled ventilation can further depress myocardial contractility. Blood loss can compromise venous return to the heart. The stress response can cause tachycardia and hypertension which compromise myocardial oxygenation.

Although the anaesthetist does his best to minimize these effects the cardiovascular system must be robust enough to withstand these potential effects on venous return and myocardial function.

Wake the patient up in a comfortable condition

Recovery from anaesthesia is in part dependent on hepatic and renal function depending on the anaesthetic drugs used. Compromise in either renal or hepatic function may affect the metabolism and elimination of drugs. Smaller doses of analgesic agents may be required. Supplementary analgesics may, however, be required in any patient during recovery.

INVESTIGATIONS

Local guidelines may be in place. The pre-operative investigation of specific diseases is dealt with in a separate chapter which covers the entire peri-operative management of those diseases.

Airway

Consider facial deformity, past surgery or conditions restricting neck movement as potential problems. Further discussion on the investigation of airway problems is beyond the scope of a gynaecology textbook. Advice should be taken from the anaesthetist e.g. X-rays or other radiological investigation of neck in rheumatoid arthritis.

Miscellaneous

A history/family history of malignant hyperpyrexia or suxamethonium apnoea must be reported to the anaesthetist as early as possible.

Assessment of spread of malignant disease

It would be expected that comprehensive assessment would have been done as part of the investigation of the disease. If there is any suspicion of metastatic disease a pre-operative chest X-ray and LFTs are indicated.

Fitness for day case anaesthesia

Local criteria may be in place.

As a general rule day case surgery should be restricted to healthy patients and those with mild systemic disease. It is acceptable to include patients with well-controlled systemic diseases such as non-insulin dependent diabetes or hypertension. The age limit is flexible and selection should depend more on fitness. Consideration must be given to supervision in the domestic environment and the availability of an escort and transport to go home.

Fasting

For elective surgery, water (maximum of an ordinary glass per hour) may be given up to 2 h before the proposed starting time of an operation. Light food may be given up to 6 h before. Fatty foods, very cold drinks, fizzy drinks and drinks containing a large amount of sugar should be avoided. Up to 60 ml of water can be allowed for swallowing of medication. For emergency surgery the patient should be kept nil by mouth from the time of admission to hospital until discussion with the anaesthetist takes place.

What do you do with the patient whose surgery is cancelled for medical reasons?

Speak to the anaesthetist to ask specifically what must be done to render the patient fit for anaesthesia e.g. consult GP, physicians, put onto senior anaesthetist's list etc. Ask how to get an early anaesthetic opinion at the time of subsequent admission to prevent the same occurring. If the reason is a serious medical problem e.g. congestive cardiac failure, unstable angina or severe hypertension, take a medical opinion before the patient is discharged. As much as possible partake in arrangement to sort out the problem and reschedule surgery as soon as possible to avoid complaint. An early phone call to the anaesthetist at the time of readmission may avoid problems.

PERI-OPERATIVE MANAGEMENT OF COMMON PRE-EXISTING DISEASES

Barry Miller and Kate Grady

For all diseases advice is given for straightforward assessment and investigation. The non-straightforward case or abnormal findings on investigation and examination should be referred to the anaesthetist.

LUNG DISEASES

Asthma

From history record when was condition diagnosed, hospital admissions, recent hospital admissions, ICU admissions, medication. On examination chest should be clear. Peak expiratory flow rate (PEFR) gives baseline information.

- Use β-agonist inhaler or nebulizer prior to theatre and consider the need for steroid cover (if recent or current oral therapy).

Chronic respiratory disease e.g. chronic bronchitis, emphysema, 'COAD'

From history record when was condition diagnosed, hospital admissions, recent hospital admissions, ICU admissions, medication, smoking, cardiovascular system (CVS) history and function. New York Heart Association (NYHA) grading system for functional dyspnoea gives a useful rule of thumb when deciding on further investigations:

Graded for shortage of breath (SOB):

1 nil;
2 on severe exertion;
3 on mild exertion;
4 at rest.

Grades 3 or 4 will warrant greater investigation and possible pre-operative admission for management.

Examination of chest often reveals scattered wheezes and crepitations. Focal areas may indicate active infection. Get chest X-ray (CXR) for all if not had one in the last 3 months, PEFR, FBC (to check WCC for active disease and exclude anaemia), U&Es (to check potassium as usually on diuretics).

If NYHA Grade 3 or 4 do arterial blood gases (to assess baseline hypoxia, and exclude CO_2 retention), lung function tests (a good assessment of poor lung function in which case operative risk needs to be qualified).

- Patients should be admitted 24 h pre-operatively and the anaesthetist alerted.
- May require in-hospital antibiotics, chest physiotherapy and oxygen to optimize.
- Consider peri-operative steroid cover.
- Regular and PRN nebulizers are more efficient and effective than the patients' own inhalers.
- Take advice on post-operative pain management to ensure adequate cough.
- Regularly assess for developing chest infections.

CARDIOVASCULAR DISEASES

From history record chest pain, palpitations, blackouts, dyspnoea or orthopnoea, hypertension and treated hypertension, diabetes mellitus, smoker, treated arrhythmias. Investigations comprise ECG in anyone over the age of 60 or with the above symptoms. For stress tests and echocardiograms take the advice of the anaesthetist.

If pacemaker *in situ*, get ECG, U&Es and details of type of pacemaker and when it was last checked.

There are four interlinked aspects that define cardiovascular disease.

1 Coronary artery disease.
2 Myocardial dysfunction.
3 Arrythmias.
4 Valvular problems.

Any one or more may be present, and any assessment should consider all four areas.

Coronary artery disease

This is the main cause of ischaemic heart disease, often leading to myocardial dysfunction and arrhythmias. Record from history chest pain (main symptom), history of MI, angioplasty or coronary artery by-pass surgery. Avoid surgery within 6 months of an MI. Assess stability of angina over last year.

Assess severity of pain (Canadian Cardiovascular Society):

1 nil;
2 mild (pain on more than one flight of stairs);
3 moderate (pain on the flat);
4 severe (pain with minimal activity or at rest).

Moderate pain or greater warrants cardiological investigation.

On examination coronary artery disease itself has few signs, although peripheral vascular disease suggests its presence.

Get ECG to exclude ischaemia at rest (compare with last ECG if available to assess stability) and arrhythmias.

Ensure good pre-medication and post-operative analgesia. Give oxygen post-operatively for 48 h. Those who have had an MI are at increased risk of ischaemic heart disease and re-infarction in the peri-operative period. The risk is associated with the presence of heart failure, increasing age, valvular disease and an operation within an abdominal cavity. Overall the risk is highest in the first 3 months (approx. 25%) and lower in the second 3 months (15%). It remains steady after 6 months at 5% (0.1% for a first event). For patients who have had an MI within the last 6 months the urgency of the procedure should be considered and the opinion of a consultant anaesthetist should be taken. For those with co-incident cardiac failure the general physicians/cardiologists should be involved.

Myocardial dysfunction

Usually due to coronary artery disease, but can be valvular. From history record evidence of heart failure i.e. dyspnoea, orthopnoea and paroxysmal nocturnal dyspnoea.

On examination assess chest basal crepitations, ankle/calf/sacral oedema. Investigations comprise:

- FBC (to exclude anaemia as this impedes myocardial oxygen delivery);

- U&Es (to exclude hypokalaemia as on diuretics and ACE inhibitors);
- CXR;
- Consider echocardiogram to assess ejection fraction if symptoms and signs marked despite treatment.

May require medical review to confirm that treatment is maximized.

Arrhythmias

- From history, record 'dizzy' spells or blackouts and whether on anticoagulants.
- Examine pulse.
- Investigations comprise FBC, U&Es, digoxin levels, clotting studies and ECG.
- All should be medically controlled pre-operatively. Even if stable, peri-operative stress may lead to CVS instability.
- Unmanaged arrhythmia needs medical advice on drugs or need for pacing. Drugs should be continued peri-operatively.
- More than 48 h of poor oral intake requires specialist advice regarding maintenance digoxin.

Valvular problems

From history record symptoms of coronary artery disease, myocardial dysfunction, arrhythmias or asymptomatic. Patient has often been told they need antibiotics when visiting the dentist. Record whether on anticoagulants.

Examination

It is often difficult to detect important diastolic murmurs.

Investigations

Depending on other symptoms and signs:

- consider CXR;
- consider echocardiogram if undefined and associated with symptoms and signs. Mandatory if suspicion of aortic stenosis.

Antibiotic prophylaxis

See BNF for latest guidelines.

HYPERTENSION

- Record angina symptoms from history.
- ECG is mandatory and check U&Es if on diuretics or ACE inhibitors.
- If diastolic pressure is >110 mmHg, recheck at least twice over the next 2 h to exclude stress-related cause (not usually this marked). If it stays >110, cancel and refer to GP. If in pre-operative clinic, refer to GP. GP should be asked to confirm normotension.
- If diastolic pressure <110, but >90 mmHg, check with the anaesthetist.
- If diastolic pressure >120 mmHg, refer to physicians for immediate opinion.

DIABETES MELLITUS

In practical terms, four aspects of the peri-operative management must be considered:

1 NIDDM – Usually seen in the middle aged or elderly, often overweight, and on oral medication;
2 IDDM – Any age group, and may include those whose NIDDM cannot be controlled with diet and oral medication;
3 Day case surgery;
4 Overnight or longer stay – especially if oral intake is compromised.

History

- Current medication: oral hypoglycaemics or insulin regimen.
- Changes over the last year.
- Hospital admissions for hypoglycaemic or diabetic ketoacidotic episodes.
- Hypoglycaemic episodes treated by patient (especially last 12 months).
- Associated disease (especially CVS, renal and autonomic).

Examination

- Weight.

Investigations

- FBC, U+Es (especially K^+), random blood sugar.
- In urgent cases with >24 h history perform arterial blood gases.

Management

- Ideally patients should be first on a morning list.

Day case

NIDDM:
- Drugs need to have been reviewed in clinic.
- Stop oral hypoglycaemics on morning of surgery, except chlorpropramide, which needs to have been stopped the day before.

IDDM:
- On morning list: omit morning insulin.
- On afternoon list: light early breakfast and insulin.
- Post-operative: home, after eating and insulin restart. If nausea and vomiting consider overnight stay and dextrose insulin potassium (DKI) regimen.

In-patient

- All patients (NIDDM and IDDM) should be started on a DKI regimen. Most hospitals have a standard one, as does the BNF.
- Start on morning of surgery – requires daily U+Es (K^+) post-operatively.

Consider:

1 Fluid load – 3 l per day may be too much in the CVS disease group.
2 ⇓ [Na^+] may require use of 4% dextose/0.18% saline or 5% dextrose/0.45% saline (available from paediatric wards, and suitable for use via a peripheral line).

Ask for early advice – poor intake post-operatively needs senior intervention.

NEUROLOGICAL DISEASES

Diseases affecting the nervous system can be considered in two basic categories.

1 Stable underling disease with fixed deficit.
2 Progressive disease.

Epilepsy

- History: When was it diagnosed? Was there a precipitating cause? How often do fits occur? What is their nature? Any changes in the last 6–12 months. Will a fit affect the patient's life – e.g. loss of driving licence.
- Medication: Anticonvulsants.
- Examination: Nil, except evidence from causative CNS lesion if present.
- Investigations: FBC (tendency for aplasia), consider LFTs if major surgery.
- Management: Continue drugs in the peri-operative period (especially day of operation).

Liaise with patient, ward staff and others about maintenance of drug therapy if NBM. Post-operatively consider PR or parenteral preps (liaise with neurologist/ physicians).

Multiple sclerosis

- History: When did it start? Any recent deteriorations? Nature of disability – contractures may make positioning difficult.
- Medication: Often symptomatic treatments.
- Examination: Assessment of disabilities – especially with relation to theatre positioning.
- Investigations: U+Es especially potassium if there is a large motor deficit.
- Management: Although there is no evidence patient should be advised of the long held feeling that surgery/anaesthesia may precipitate a relapse. The same is true for regional blockade; the anaesthetist should discuss this with the patient.

Motor neurone disease (MND)

As for MS, but consider potential post-operative respiratory complications – assess as for RS disease.

Myotonias

As for MND, but also consider cardiomyopathies – assess as for CVS disease (especially myocardial dysfunction).

RHEUMATOID ARTHRITIS AND OTHER CONNECTIVE TISSUE DISEASES

This is a multisystem condition. Consider respiratory and cardiovascular symptoms and pay attention to the involvement of neck and temperomandibular joints. Record whether hip or knee involvement as this affects positioning.

- Medication: Often complex: doses and days of medication should be noted. In general, continue all drugs, and provide cover for steroids. Check for maximum steroid dose in the last 3 months.

- Investigation: FBC – often low Hb, but check for low WCC. U+Es (especially if on immunosuppressive drugs – methotrexate, gold, cyclosporin). CXR and ECG if directed. Consider neck views in liaison with Anaesthetist and Radiologist, maintenance of medication, and appropriate steroid cover. Caution with joint movement, especially under anaesthetic.

THYROID DISEASE

- From history record is the patient euthyroid? When was it last checked? – remember that if you want a result, tests are usually performed monthly by most laboratories. List appropriately. Has patient been told of a retrosternal goitre? Whether on therapy and whether therapy stable.
- Examine to exclude thyroid gland size: Is there a goitre?
- Check pulse – HR is a good indication of hypo-/hyper-thyroid function.
- Investigation: Check for most recent TFTs – consider thoracic inlet views – for retrosternal goitre, check with anaesthetist. Continue medication pre-operatively.

LIVER DISEASE

- History: Length of disease. Possible causes – most commonly viral hepatitis or alcohol.
- Associated problems: CVS (secondary to fluid balance problems) and immuno-suppression
- Consider Physician review – is condition optimized?
- Examination: Ascites, peripheral oedema, liver and spleen palpation. Jaundice is a relatively rare, and late sign.
- Medication: Often minimal, aim to keep it that way. Spironolactone – Check K$^+$.
- Investigation: FBC, clotting (consider G+S), U+Es, LFTs (mainly for total protein and albumin levels).
- Management: Consider Vitamin K and availability of FFP for surgery – even laparoscopic work risks major haemorrhage if a vessel is damaged. Propensity to develop hypoglycaemia – consider early in any post-operative confusion. Avoid im injections – consider Vitamin K, by iv infusion and post-operative analgesia by oral or iv medication.
- Caution with iv opioids.

RENAL DISEASE

- From history record whether on dialysis or whether had transplant.
- Examine for peripheral oedema, pulmonary oedema, hypertension.
- Investigation: FBC (Hb often low): Consider need for post/intra-operative transfusion, clotting – if regional anaesthesia considered. U+Es especially potassium in all those on diuretic therapy, in diabetes, acute abdomen, if iv fluids or nil by mouth or having nasogastric aspiration, LFTs – albumin level. Consider CXR and ECG, if systems affected.
- Consider best timing for pre- and post-operative dialysis (practicalities of latter). Caution with fluid, Na$^+$ and K$^+$ intake (Consider insensible losses – may be very small or very great). Liaise with anaesthetist and physicians.

- Consider invasive monitoring if large post-operative fluid shifts. Daily U+Es are essential. Patient may benefit from regional anaesthesia/analgesia. If poor renal function – caution with drugs – e.g. Morphine as half-life may be prolonged – avoid further risk to renal function – e.g. NSAIDs.

PERI-OPERATIVE MANAGEMENT OF REGULAR MEDICATION

Barry Miller and Kate Grady

RESPIRATORY DRUGS

ACTION PLAN

1 All drugs should be continued in the peri-operative period

Inhalers
Supplement with regular and/or as required nebulizers.

Oxygen
Oxygen is often needed in the peri-operative period. It should not be restricted to 28% or less, without evidence of Type 2 respiratory failure and CO_2 retention. The latter is usually a function of exhaustion requiring more O_2 not less. If you feel oxygen restriction is appropriate discuss with anaesthetist.

Steroids
Therapy should be continued but may need to convert to parenteral.

CARDIOVASCULAR DRUGS

ACTION PLAN

1 In general, drugs needed to treat hypertension, ischaemic heart disease and control arrhythmias should be continued peri-operatively

β-blockers
Check pulse rate and ECG rate. Usually continued but discuss with anaesthetist, especially if heart rate <50/min and/or arrhythmia.

Diuretics
Check U&Es especially potassium. Wide variation in practice but potassium-sparing diuretics e.g. amiloride are usually omitted.

ACE inhibitors
Check U&Es especially potassium. Wide variation in practice but usually omitted.

Anti-arrhythmics
Continue. Check ECG, U&Es especially potassium to exclude electrolyte abnormality as cause of intra-operative arrhythmia.
Check digoxin level. Will need baseline if oral intake of digoxin precluded.

Aspirin
Whether to continue is a consideration of balance between bleeding intra- and post-operatively and the risk of thromboembolism. Continuation of aspirin should also be discussed with anaesthetist as there are variable opinions with regard to the relative contraindication of regional blocks in those taking aspirin. If it is to be stopped this has to be 7 days before surgery to be effective.

DIABETES MELLITUS TREATMENT

1 Oral hypoglycaemics
- Sulphonoureas e.g. glicazide and glibencalmide should be stopped on day of surgery. The exception is chlorpropramide which should be stopped on the day before surgery.
- Metformin should be stopped on day of surgery – if patient becomes ill, early arterial blood gases will help to exclude lactic acidosis.

2 Insulin
- Majority of patients will convert easily to a standard dextrose/insulin/potassium (DKI) regimen (If >100 u/day of insulin seek specialist advice.).
- Modified from the BNF guidelines:
  1 The basic aim is for 5–10 g glucose/hour to be infused, and the blood glucose level to be controlled with insulin.
  2 Serum [K+] is particularly at risk of severe variation, and so it should be checked pre-operatively. If not hyperkalaemic, K+ should be added to the infusate at 10 mmol/l.
  3 A suitable regimen would run:
     - 10% glucose solution, with [K+] 10 mmol/l run at 100–125 ml/h.
     - Insulin solution: Soluble insulin 1 unit/ml made up in 0.9% saline in a 50 ml syringe.
     - The two infusions should run through the same iv cannula, preventing the solo administration of one drug if cannula failure occurs.
     - A pre-operative fasting glucose is measured and the insulin infusion started.

Blood glucose	Insulin: units/h
<3	Stop insulin
4	0.5
5–15	2
16–20	4
>21	Call senior assistance

Blood glucose is measured hourly until stable, and then 2 hourly.

Helpful hints:
1 The basic principle is to avoid ketoacidosis, by a continuous supply of glucose and insulin.
2 If fluid volume is critical, consider that 1 g glucose is 10 ml of 10% glucose solution or 20 ml 5% glucose solution.
3 If [Na+] is an issue use a glucose/saline solution. Although 4% glucose/0.18% saline is the most commonly available on UK adult wards, 5% glucose/0.45% saline is available on most paediatric wards and is better for [Na+] control. (Consider that an equal infusion rate of 10% glucose and 0.9% saline is the same thing, but multiple bags of fluid are difficult to monitor, and are best avoided.)
4 Any of the above solutions should have [K+] added, as appropriate.
5 It is possible to have all the drugs in one bag (insulin, glucose, potassium), however, with modern infusion devices these systems ('Alberti regimes') are used less frequently due to their high labour intensiveness. The use of sc insulin is to be avoided.

EPILEPSY DRUGS

1 If considering infertility treatment give folate supplements 5 mg/day (to reduce chance of neural tube defect) and liaise with neurologist/GP to reduce number of anticonvulsants if taking more than one

2 Check FBC and for longer procedures check LFTs and clotting

3 Abnormalities should be reviewed by anaesthetist/physician before elective surgery

WARFARIN

This is a complex area, and early discussion with both the haematologist and anaesthetist is necessary. The time consuming need for careful adjustment from oral to parenteral control means that elective admission on the day or the previous day should not be done without a documented plan. Such a plan should be drawn up at the out-patient stage.

1 It is essential to know why the patient is on warfarin and what INR is being aimed for

2 Check INR, APTT ratio and FBC.

3 The overall management advice can be taken as (British Committee for Standards in Haematology):

- (Minor) surgery – with little intra- or post-operative bleeding risk can be performed with an INR<2.5.
- Majority of surgery needs an INR<1.5.

The management should be discussed with the haematologist but for major surgery usually stop warfarin 3–4 days pre-operatively and start unfractionated heparin iv infusion (~30 000 units/day) the next day.

Aim for APTT ratio 1.5–2.5. Stop 6 hours pre-operatively. Check INR and APTT 1 hour pre-operatively. Re-start 12 hours post-operatively. Haematological advice may suggest the use of the low molecular weight heparins, with or without specific monitoring. A discussion of such advice is beyond the scope of this chapter.

4 Other considerations with warfarin:

- Mechanical prosthetic heart valves: Variable practice – general rules apply. Current opinion (*Brit. J. Haem.* 1998 **101:** 374 – 387) suggests that 'the short term risk of thromboembolism in patients with mechanical heart valves when not anticoagulated is very small, <0.2% over a 7 day period'.
- Treated deep vein thrombosis: This is usually treated for 3–6 months. If possible, surgery should be avoided until 1 month after anticoagulation is no longer required. If it is not possible to delay for that length of time, consider a standard regimen.

- Emergency surgery: Discuss with anaesthetist and haematologist. Check INR and FBC. Consider fresh frozen plasma (FFP; 10–15 ml/kg) – Recheck INR.
- IV Vitamin K (1–2 mg) may be used but makes post-operative anticoagulation difficult.

PERI-OPERATIVE STEROID COVER

ACTION PLAN

1 **Ongoing steroid therapy causes suppression of the hypothalamic-pituitary-adrenal axis and prevents the production of steroid hormones as part of the natural stress response. The past practice of prolonged high dose cover, has now been modified, as it has been recognized that excessive peri-operative steroid therapy is as much a potential problem, as under-treatment**

2 **Consider**
- Normal body cortisol production ~ 25 mg/day.
- Stress response up to ~100 mg/day.
- Cortisol 1 mg = Hydrocortisone 1 mg.

3 **History**
- Has the patient been on steroids in the last 3 months – Treat as for highest dose in that time.
- Has the dose been stable over the last 3 months?
  If not:
  1 Is the patient currently on a reducing dose? Treat as for maximum dose in the last 3 months.
  2 Is the current dose a treatment for exacerbation of the underlying disease? – Consider postponing the procedure, or treat as for current dose.
  3 Is the dose for 'immunosuppressive' purposes?

4 **Convert drug to hydrocortisone equivalents**

Hydrocortisone 20 mg =

Prednisolone   5 mg
Dexamethosone   750 µg
MethylPrednisolone 4 mg

(See BNF for a complete discussion.)

10–25 mg/day prednisolone:

Mod. Surgery:	Pre-operative dose + 25 mg hydrocortisone at induction + 100 mg/day** for 24 h (Return to pre-operative oral, or iv equivalent)
Major Surgery:	Pre-operative dose + 25 mg hydrocortisone at induction +100 mg/day** for 48–72h (Return to pre-operative oral, or iv equivalent)

Appendix 1

218

| >100 mg/day (immunosuppressive) | Convert to iv equivalent in the peri-operative period until oral intake recommenced |
| >25 mg/day prednisolone | No additional steroid necessary |

[** 100 mg/day either as a continuous infusion, or as 25–50 mg 6–12 hourly]

LARGE DOSE OPIOIDS

1 **Seek specialist advice from the anaesthetist and/or the pain service**
- Patients will have both a tolerance to these doses and withdrawal symptoms if stopped precipitously. The concept of dependency is a complex psychosocial entity – based around drug seeking behaviour, and not relevant here.

2 **Routine drugs (e.g. methadone, MST, fentanyl patches) should be continued throughout the peri-operative period**

3 **The provision of analgesia for the acute pain of surgery often necessitates the use of large doses of opioids. These doses often alarm medical and nursing staff**

4 **Doses should be calculated around the baseline drug**
- Calculate a 24 h oral morphine equivalent.
- Consider that 'breakthrough' pain is treated at ~ 1/5 to 1/6 of the full daily dose.
- Consider that the parenteral dose is ~ 1/2 to 1/3 of the oral.
- PCA (in addition) to the baseline drug is often sufficient.

Example:
Fentanyl patch 125 μg/h.
Oral morphine equivalent ~ 450 mg/24 h.
Oral breakthrough dose ~ 75–90 mg (can be given 2 hourly).
Parenteral equivalent: 25–45 mg morphine.

Most PCA systems will happily deliver 1 mg morphine with a 5 min lockout, 12 mg in an hour.

Although the initial analgesia may require a large bolus, maintenance rarely then requires much intervention.

5 **If analgesia is inadequate specialist advice of pain team should be sought and analgesia established by iv bolus. The dose should then be increased, and the lockout maintained**

6 **Regular (not PRN) addition of paracetamol (PO or PR) and, where tolerant, a regular NSAID (PO or PR) will help reduce the dose of PRN opioid in most patients**

COMBINED ORAL CONTRACEPTIVE PILL (COCP) AND HORMONE REPLACEMENT THERAPY (HRT)

ACTION PLAN

1 The COCP should be stopped 4–6 weeks before major surgery. This is not necessary for minor surgery

2 Alternative contraceptive arrangements need to be discussed at the time that surgery is recommended

3 When this is not possible as in emergency surgery thromboprophylaxis and graduated compression stockings should be used

4 HRT does not need to be stopped but thromboprohylaxis should be given

THYROID DISEASE

ACTION PLAN

1 The most important factor is that the patient is euthyroid and stable

2 For replacement therapy: Continue, consider TFTs if clinically hypothyroid

3 For anti-thyroid drugs: Continue, need FBC pre-operatively as small agranulocytosis risk. Recent evidence of a stable euthyroid state should be checked, and TFTs considered (remember the results may take up to a month)

4 β-blockers as for CVS indication

PSYCHIATRIC MEDICATION

ACTION PLAN

1 Antidepressants: Most should be continued. Monoamineoxidase inhibitors (MAOIs), even the newer reversible ones, should preferably be stopped at least 2–3 weeks before surgery, and suitable replacement therapy instituted. This will require liaison with the GP and/or psychiatrist as this patient must have a serious depression to be taking such a drug. If this is not possible, e.g. emergency surgery it should be brought to the attention of the anaesthetist. Post-operative analgesia should be discussed with the anaesthetist and pethidine must be avoided

2 Anti-psychotics: Usually continued

3 Lithium: Discuss with anaesthetist, as there is wide variation in practice. It is usually discontinued 24–48 h before major surgery. Check U&Es and [Li+] (therapeutic levels 0.4–1.0 mmol/l). Lithium toxicity is potentiated by low [Na+], a particular risk if diuretics are also being taken

H$_2$ ANTAGONISTS AND PROTON PUMP INHIBITORS

ACTION PLAN

1 Continue

PERI-OPERATIVE MANAGEMENT OF FLUID AND ELECTROLYTE BALANCE

Barry Miller and Kate Grady

Peri-operative fluid balance is seen as complex but need not be so if a few basic rules are adopted. The first is to take note of the fluid history, as determined by the features of the patient's illness and peri-operative course. Fluid balance is an on-going process and starts or dates back to the time when normal oral intake stopped. Variation in fluid prescription is as important as the changes in insulin requirements in the diabetic patient. In all but the simplest cases, regular and *frequent* assessments are needed.

Fluids

Output:

- Insensible loss 0.5 ml/kg/h = 780 ml (45% lungs and 55% skin).
  This value will increase by ~12% per 1°C temperature increase.
- Urine 0.5 – 1.0 ml/kg/h.

Thus, hourly loss, in normal circumstances is ~ 1.5 ml/kg/h. A good rule of thumb peri-operatively is 2–3 ml/kg/h. Remember to back calculate.

Replacement may need to be greater than this depending on surgical factors such as the development of ileus and blood loss. Losses relating to the peri-operative period are, obviously, the most difficult to estimate, but consider the following short list as a basic framework.

- Losses from an open body cavity ~ 5 ml/kg/h (intra-operative).
- Losses relating to blood loss – This may be a major issue in either the pre-operative or post-operative period.
- '3rd Space' losses: This is the most nebulous area of all, but relates mainly to fluid sequestered in the GI tract – usually as a consequence of intestinal stasis – and oedema of the abdominal contents due to sepsis, handling or trauma during surgery.

Electrolytes

Major daily shifts are of water Na, K and toxins

Na$^+$ and K$^+$ daily input are both ~ 1 mmol/kg. But remember there may be electrolyte disturbances in the peri-operative period so be guided by the regular U&Es:

- Plasma [Na$^+$] = 140 +/− 0.5 mmol/l.
- Plasma [K$^+$] = 4.0 +/− 0.5 mmol/l.

Cardiovascular (CVS) parameters

Heart rate and blood pressure are very easy to measure, and notoriously difficult to interpret. The body's compensatory mechanisms are very efficient, and so the simple measures available on most wards must be viewed critically. The first important rule is that absolute values in the 'normal' range are pretty meaningless. Their importance lies in *relative* changes, and *trends*, e.g. HR 60 with BP 140/75, and HR 85 with BP 120/60.

Both these sets of values are 'normal', but a change from the first to the second, needs careful review.

Except in the case of rapid haemorrhage, gross changes in CVS values are rarely encountered until a substantial fluid deficit in one or more body compartment has occurred.

Hourly urine output is a very valuable measure of fluid balance, and should be considered early in any patient with potential or known fluid balance problems. Normal output is around 1 ml/kg/h. Oliguria is usually defined as the production of less than 0.5 ml/kg/h. This will be recognized in 2 or 3 h in the catheterized patient, but may not be noticed in the non-catheterized patient for 12 or even 24 hours.

Central venous pressure (CVP) measurement is useful in this area as trends relating to intravascular fluid volume are more easily assessed. However, in practice, the continual measurement of the CVP is rarely available on most ordinary wards. There are difficulties both in the siting of the line, and its management, which must be addressed.

Other factors

Skin turgor and mucous membranes are rarely of practical value, however, the sensation, and verbalization, of thirst is a very useful indicator of fluid deficit, when present.

Simple management

The first rule in any management plan is to 'Know your Tools'. There are a variety of fluids available, and each has distinct physiological properties best employed for specific tasks.

Crystalloids

This refers to any simple solution that passes through a semi-permeable membrane. The most common available are:

- 0.9% ('Normal') saline: [Na$^+$] 154 mmol/l. This fluid causes expansion only of the ECF. The volume of infused fluid needed to replace haemorrhagic losses is about 3x the estimated loss.
- Compound sodium lactate (Hartmann's/Ringer's): Properties essentially as for 0.9% saline.
- 5% dextrose: this fluid expands throughout the total body water, about one third remains in the ECF, and about one quarter in the intravascular space (IVS).
- Glucose/saline mixtures:
  4% dextrose/0.18% saline : 7/15th enters the ECF.
  5% dextrose/0.45% saline : 2/3rd remain in ECF.

Colloids

This refers to a suspension of particles rather than a solution, unable to pass through a semi-permeable membrane. Because of this property they tend to stay in the IVS, and are often termed 'Plasma expanders':

- Gelatin derivatives – effect on the IVS is only a few hours. Some contain Ca$^+$ and will require a change of giving set before blood is given.
- Hetastarch/Pentastarch – effects on the IVS may be for 24 hours or more. Most commonly used in ITU situations.

- Blood products:
    1. Albumin – rarely used except in children and under specialist advice.
    2. Blood – most commonly as 'packed cells': Will need additional crystalloid or colloid when used for acute haemorrhage.
    3. Dextrans – may affect coagulation, blood cross matching and kidney function. Rarely used now in the UK, except in specialist circumstances.

PERI-OPERATIVE MANAGEMENT OF THE EARLY PREGNANT PATIENT

Kate Grady and Barry Miller

ANAESTHESIA IN EARLY PREGNANCY

If possible, exposure to drugs and surgery should be avoided during pregnancy. When a procedure is necessary, the risks must be minimized. Early discussion between anaesthetist and surgeon allows review of the risks and options and time for counselling and appropriate pre-medication.

The problems are:

- Increased risk of anaesthesia to mother in pregnancy.
- Drug effects on the fetus.
- Risk of abortion.

Increased risk of anaesthesia to mother in pregnancy

The increased risks are of aspiration and of exacerbation of an underlying condition.

Aspiration

One of the perennial risks in anaesthesia is that of aspiration of stomach contents. Gastric motility and oesophageal sphincter tone are reduced in pregnancy. This occurs early in the first trimester, and is worsened by the physical displacement of by the enlarging uterus in later pregnancy.

Two options may be considered.

- Avoid the use of a GA, where possible – this may also be useful in reducing the drugs exposed to the fetus.
- Consider the use of prokinetics and / or H_2-antagonists. As in obstetric anaesthesia, the use of sodium citrate immediately pre-operatively is often used.

Structural heart problems

Although many conditions improve under pregnancy – probably as a result of hormonal variations – structural heart conditions often worsen. Although much rarer now than 50 years ago, mainly due to the disappearance of rheumatic heart disease, the survival of individuals with congenital heart problems, with or without a history of surgery or medications is increasingly common.

It is not possible to detail the problems here, but any patient with a known problem should be discussed early. The history must concentrate on the changes from the pre-pregnancy state (often from no symptoms to quite severe ones). *See chapter on preoperative assessment.*

Investigations should include:

- FBC – Although physiological anaemia is normal, toleration of low Hb levels may be poor and require transfusion. Care must be taken with the infused load.
- ECG – Evidence of rhythm, strain and even ischaemia.
- Echocardiography – Evidence of functional deficits can be assessed.

The latter two are particularly useful if pre- or early pregnancy readings were known.

Drug effects on the fetus

The safe use of drugs during pregnancy is a continuing problem. Few drugs have a clear licence, and this is likely to remain so for the foreseeable future. The largest problem arises with new drugs, whose overall profiles are often good but for which stringent recommendations often preclude their usage. In any specialist field, the use of medication must be directed by specialist literature. The potential for teratogenicity is greatest in the first trimester, although present throughout pregnancy. (The BNF has a very good guide on drugs in pregnancy, and their trimester-related risks. Specialist advice should always be sought on unfamiliar drugs or prolonged prescription.)

The basic rule should be, the fewer the drugs, and the lower the dosages, the better'. To this end, the use of local or regional techniques is often preferred. Although with local infiltration, consideration must be given to the total amount of local anaesthetic given. The details of a GA will depend on the planned procedure and time should be available for maternal counselling. Because of the ethics of research in pregnancy there are no controlled studies in pregnant women. The drugs which are used are ones in which animal studies have failed to demonstrate a fetal risk or have shown an adverse effect that was not confirmed in controlled studies in women in the first trimester.

Drugs for which there is positive evidence of human fetal risk and likelihood of causing fetal abnormalities outweighs any benefit should be avoided.

Paracetamol: There are no reports of congenital abnormalities attributed to Paracetamol. Fetal death has been reported in maternal overdose.

Aspirin and NSAIDs: The use of these drugs in the third trimester is associated with premature closure of the ductus arteriosus. There is a risk of neonatal haemorrhage. Low dose NSAIDs in the second trimester are associated with oligohydramnios. The above risks do not appear to apply to low dose aspirin as used in pre-eclampsia.

Opioids: Use of codeine in the first trimester is associated with respiratory malformations, congenital heart disease and cleft lip and palate. In the first and second trimesters it is associated with inguinal and umbilical hernias and a neonatal withdrawal syndrome is described.

Dextropropoxyphene is associated with a neonatal withdrawal syndrome. Morphine is safely used for short-term interventions. Most of the available long-term data is for methadone which is associated with good maternal and fetal outcome.

Consideration should also be given to appropriate and effective anti-emetics. First choice should probably be an antihistamine (e.g. cyclizine), and second line a phenothiazine (e.g. prochlorperazine).

The use of epidural infusions (of local anaesthetic ± opioid may also be appropriate. Good analgesia is important, to help reduce stress responses, a factor in abortion (see below).

Risk of abortion

The cause of most abortions is unknown. Although, suspicion has fallen on some anaesthetic drugs (most notably halothane and nitrous oxide) a link has never been established (suggesting that even if present, it is very small). The most common risks seen in this situation are cardiovascular instability and systemic illness especially sepsis. Appropriate use of fluids, O_2 and analgesics should help to minimize these.

Drugs must be carefully selected and attention given to the timing of the fetus's exposure to the drug. The dose and duration of exposure should be minimized.

PERI-OPERATIVE MANAGEMENT OF PATIENT DECLINING BLOOD AND BLOOD PRODUCTS

Kate Grady

Patients, regardless of religious belief may decline the use of blood and blood products for many reasons. Jehovah's Witnesses believe that blood transfusion is forbidden. This is a deeply held core value and they regard a non-consensual transfusion as a gross physical violation. Witnesses view scripture as ruling out transfusion of whole blood, packed red blood cells, white blood cells, plasma, and platelets. Witnesses' religious understanding does not absolutely prohibit the use of minor blood fractions such as clotting factors. Jehovah's witnesses are not 'anti-medicine' and wish to be treated with effective non-blood medical alternatives to allogeneic blood. A doctor is obliged to give the best care to his patient in keeping with the patient's wishes. He should be aware of the patient's specific wishes and do his best to comply with these. All members of the gynaecology (and theatre if appropriate) team should be made aware of the situation and of the care/contingency plan should haemorrhage occur. The patient's wishes and discussions should be clearly documented.

1 Attend to issues of consent

- To administer blood in the face of refusal by a competent adult patient is unlawful.
- Ensure that the patient has had the opportunity to speak with the gynaecologist in privacy, without relatives or members of her religious community if she wishes.
- Keep a clear record of discussion and particular aspects of consent.
- Note precisely which products/treatment (e.g. cell savers) she refuses and which she would accept. Complete a Jehovah's Witness consent form.
- Have discussion and take and document consent in the presence of a witness. If in the case of severe haemorrhage, a further surgical procedure would be contemplated this should be discussed and consented for.
- The person witnessing the discussion should sign a record of the discussion and consent as made and signed by the doctor.
- A verbally expressed change of mind should be honoured. Again it should be given in the presence of a witness and recorded in the notes.
- Allow the patient the opportunity to speak with the Hospital Liaison Committee for Jehovah's Witnesses and if requested join their discussion.

If the patient is a minor, parental right to determine whether or not she will have medical treatment terminates if she has sufficient understanding and intelligence to enable her to comprehend fully what is proposed. The wishes of a competent child may be overruled if in the opinion of the court the consequences of refusal are such that it would be inappropriate to comply with the child's wishes. If the patient is too young to comprehend adequately and the parent refuses to agree to treatment that is in the opinion of qualified medical practitioners, proper and necessary, the matter can be referred to the High Court. The High Court has emergency procedures to arrange for expedited considerations of such applications. If the child is likely to succumb without the immediate administration of blood and the courts will be too time consuming blood should be transfused without consulting the court. The patient and the parents must be kept informed of proposals.

Most Jehovah's Witnesses will carry with them a clear Advance Directive prohibiting blood transfusions and will have executed a Healthcare Advance Directive which gives comprehensive personal instructions on a variety of issues. Healthcare Advanced Directives may be lodged with their GP as well as family and friends.

If the patient is not in a condition to give or withhold consent, but has previously expressed a wish at an earlier date (Advance Directive or Healthcare Advance Directive), respect the patient's instructions in the Advance Directive or Healthcare Advance Directive.

If such instructions do not specifically apply to the patient's current condition or if the patient's instructions are vague and open to interpretation or if there is good reason to believe that the patient has had a change of heart since making the declaration, the doctor's duty is to exercise good medical judgement and treat the patient in her best interests as determined by a responsible body of medical opinion.

2 Treat pre-operative anaemia

3 Reduce the risk of bleeding. Senior medical staff should be involved in care so the best of skills are employed and haemostasis must be meticulous

- The advice of the consultant haematologist should be sought in the treatment of disseminated intravascular coagulation (DIC).
- In the post-operative period monitor for bleeding so early intervention can be undertaken. After discharge from hospital the patient should have a lower threshold for seeking medical help for bleeding and should be given appropriate advice.

4 Stop blood loss

- Be vigilant in the assessment of blood loss. If stemmed early there is less risk of coagulopathy and therefore a reduced risk of further loss.
- Consider fibrinolytic inhibitors e.g. tranexamic acid and aprotinin, cryoprecipitate, Vitamin K, desmopressin.

5 Optimize other physiological variables to reduce the effect of blood loss

Some patients may accept the technique of allowing the patient to bleed into a blood tranfusion bag (available from hospital blood bank), but the blood must not lose contact with their own circulation; the intravascular volume is then replaced with clear fluid. If the patient bleeds intra-operatively it is therefore diluted blood which is lost and the blood which has been reserved in the bag immediately before surgery can then be put back into the circulation. This technique may be acceptable to some as contact is not lost with patient's own circulation. Autologous transfusion of pre-deposited blood is not an accepted technique generally. Cell savers are an accepted technique and are sometimes available on loan from Jehovah's Witness support groups. Give volume to treat hypovolaemia in the form of synthetic colloids and crystalloids. Use vasoconstrictors to maintain blood pressure. Give oxygen to optimize oxygen delivery. If very anaemic consider ventilation to optimize oxygen delivery. Start iron replacement and/or recombinant human erythropoietin. Hyperbaric treatment may be an option.

REFERENCES

Code of Practice for the Surgical Management of Jehovah's Witnesses. Royal College of Surgeons of England. London, 1996.

Management of Anaesthesia for Jehovah's Witnesses. Association of Anaesthetists of Great Britain and Ireland. London, 1999.

Treating Jehovah's Witnesses in Obstetric and Gynaecology Departments. The Hospital Liaison Committee for Jehovah's Witnesses.

USEFUL TELEPHONE NUMBER

Hospital Information Services (Britain): 020 8906 2211

Appendix 1

229

POST-OPERATIVE PAIN

Kate Grady

1 **Check observations**
   - If heart rate is increased is it due to pain, hypovolaemia or sepsis?
   - Examine further to find out.
   - Exclude hypovolaemia (increased heart rate, narrowed pulse pressure and hypotension which is a late sign).
   - Check for blood loss.
   - Exclude sepsis (unlikely) in which pulse pressure is narrowed.

2 **If severe pain (> 3/10) quickly exclude untoward surgical event, call anaesthetist and prepare for him to give 1–2 mg morphine iv, and over next 2 minutes watch for respiratory depression (RR < 8/min) or somnolence. If neither and pain uncontrolled repeat, reassess and repeat as advised by the anaesthetist**

   Anaesthetist may decide on a bolus as large as 5 mg iv. Use pulse oximetry if available (normal SaO_2 > 94%).

   Bolus should be pre-determined carefully and given slowly as do not want to have recourse to naloxone because it will reverse all analgesia and leave pain uncontrolled and even more difficult to treat. If allergic to morphine or it is contraindicated give pethidine 10–20 mg iv. Some believe morphine should be avoided in renal compromise. Do not use the im route for severe pain.

   Abdominal hysterectomy would usually require no more than 15 mg morphine in the immediate post-operative period (1 hour after gaining consciousness) if fentanyl 1 µg/kg, NSAID and morphine given intra-operatively. Requirement greater than this may point to an intra-abdominal problem.

   Laparoscopy would usually require no more than 10 mg morphine in immediate post-operative period if fentanyl 1 µg/kg and NSAID given intra-operatively.

   - Consider background infusion 1–2 mg/h of iv morphine.
   - If surgical event excluded and pain still uncontrolled call acute pain team.

   The patient on large dose strong opioids (for cancer usually) or the opioid addicted patient may have physiological tolerance and therefore need higher doses. For cancer patients on large doses of opioid take advice from the acute pain or palliative care teams, who will calculate equivalent doses for different routes and take into account post-operative pain superimposed on background pain. Strong opioids are morphine, diamorphine, fentanyl, oxycodone.

   Advice from a specialist in substance abuse is suggested for the opioid abuser.

3 **If mild (< 4/10) and able to take oral medication give oral codeine (30–60 mg) and paracetamol (1 g) together or as combination preparation. If unable to take oral give paracetamol 1 g pr**

4 **If respiratory depression occurs give naloxone 0.1–0.4 mg iv**

5 With anaesthetist decide on suitable maintenance analgesia. For a major operation this is likely to be a PCA

6 Supplement PCA with NSAID and paracetamol regularly (PR if necessary)

POST-OPERATIVE NAUSEA AND VOMITING

Kate Grady and Ilan Lieberman

Nausea and vomiting and pain are patients' greatest peri-operative concerns. The overall incidence of post-operative nausea and vomiting (PONV) is estimated at 25–30%; it is higher in gynaecological surgery. Uncontrolled PONV can have significant physiological and medical consequences and lead to delayed discharge in day case surgery.

1 **Assess for risk factors and if patient has several, discuss prophylaxis with anaesthetist. (All gynaecology patients have two risk factors!)**
   Prophylactic anti-emetics are frequently given intra-operatively. If they are to be given as a pre-medication the options are metoclopramide 10 mg po/im or cyclizine 50 mg po/im.
   Risk factors are previous PONV (3× increase), female (2–3× increase), gynaecological surgery, non-smoking, history of travel sickness, history of migraine, length of operation. There is a correlation between increasing age and decrease in PONV. Patients of twice their ideal body weight have a higher incidence after operations of longer than 3 hours.
   Of four predictors, history of motion sickness or previous PONV, female, non-smoking and use of post-operative opioids, when 0, 1, 2, 3, 4 of these were present incidence of PONV was 10, 21, 39, 61 and 79%, respectively.

2 **Ensure adequate hydration**
   Orthostatic hypotension secondary to dehydration contributes to PONV. This may be a factor in those undergoing short procedures for whom it is thought iv fluid infusion is unnecessary. Consider iv fluids for day case surgery. This is a factor in regional anaesthesia in particular.

3 **Ensure adequate pain control as pain is a major cause of PONV especially when the pain is visceral or pelvic in origin**

4 **Consider reversible causes such as hypoxia or hypoperfusion, uraemia, electrolyte disturbance, pregnancy and unstable diabetes as potential causes**
   Follow ABCs. If possible remove tactile stimulation of posterior pharynx e.g. oropharyngeal airway.
   PONV is likely to be contributed to by opioids and may be caused by other drugs e.g. syntocinon, antibiotics. More sinister causes include raised intracranial pressure, cerebral irritation e.g. infection, labyrinthine problems.

5 **Give prochloperazine 12.5 mg im or 3–6 mg buccal. If nausea controlled continue im dose 8 hourly buccal dose 12 hourly as required**

6 **If still nauseated/vomiting after 1 hour give cyclizine 50 mg im. If nausea controlled continue 8 hourly as required**

7 **If still nauseated/vomiting after 1 hour give ondansetron 4 mg iv. If nausea controlled continue cyclizine 50 mg po/im 8 hourly as required**

8 **If still nauseated/vomiting after 1 hour repeat ondasetron 4 mg iv**

9 **If PONV continues restart cycle and take advice of acute pain team**

10 **Consider non-pharmacological adjuncts. Reassurance, avoidance of excessive movement in nursing and transfer and peppermint oil may help. Acupressure has been used for prevention**

APPENDIX 2

The action plans provided in Appendix 2 direct the management of the emergency by the gynaecologist until the arrival of the medical SpR or other relevant help. In all cases, 'follow A,B,C' means:

Airway
- Assess.
- Maintain patency.
- Apply oxygen 15 l/min via tight fitting face mask with reservoir bag.
- Attach pulse oximeter to patient.

Breathing
- Assess.
- Ventilate.
- Consider intubation if hypoxic.
- Protect airway.

Circulation
- Assess pulse, BP and note for bounding peripheral pulses and warm extremities.
- CPR.
- Put on ECG and automatic NIBP monitor.
- Treat peri-arrest arrhythmias.
- iv access, send bloods (listed specifically within action plans).
- Treat hypotension.

CARDIOPULMONARY RESUSCITATION

Kate Grady

Patient appears lifeless. There is loss of consciousness, no breathing and no circulation.

1 **Ensure safe environment for victim and rescuer(s)**

2 **Shake and shout, 'Are you all right?'**

3 **If patient responds**
- Send for help if necessary.
- Assess breathing, pulse and BP.
- Regularly reassess.

4 **If no response, get help. If alone, call help before attending to patient**

5 **Open airway by head tilt, chin lift and assess breathing for 10 seconds**
- Look for chest movements.
- Listen for breath sounds.
- Feel for the movement of air.

6 **If breathing**
- Put in recovery position and ensure help on the way if necessary.
- Assess breathing, pulse and BP.
- Regularly reassess.

7 **If not breathing**
- Ensure help is on its way.
- Turn patient onto back.
- Open airway.
- Remove any obstruction from patient's mouth.

8 **Give two rescue breaths. Make no more than five attempts to achieve two breaths; if unsuccessful move on to...**

9 **Assess for signs of circulation for no more than 10 seconds**
- Look for any movement including swallowing or breathing.
- Check the carotid pulse (trained personnel).

10 **If circulation present but no breathing continue rescue breathing at a rate of 10 breaths/min. Recheck the presence of circulation every 10 breaths**

11 **If no circulation start chest compressions after two initial breaths**
- Perform 15 chest compressions.
- Continue this cycle of two breaths to 15 chest compressions.
- Compressions should be about 100/minute.

12 **If automated external defibrillator available turn to Automated External Defibrillation Algorithm on page 235**

13 **Continue until signs of life or help arrives to provide Advanced Life Support**
- Only stop to check for circulation if patient makes a movement or takes a spontaneous breath.

14 **Ensure cardiac arrest team on their way**

15 **Attach defibrillator/monitor and assess cardiac rhythm**

16 **Turn immediately to Advanced Life Support (ALS) algorithm on page 236**
- Each step that follows in the ALS algorithm assumes that the preceding one has been unsuccessful.
- Adrenaline/epinephrine 1 mg iv should be given.
- Cardiovascular collapse due to bupivacaine toxicity requires prolonged resuscitation and the use of amiodarone 300 mg.

17 **Consider and treat cause of cardiac arrest**

18 **Keep record chart of events and treatments**

19 **Record in notes and report to consultant. Inform coroner if necessary**

ALGORITHM FOR THE USE OF AUTOMATED EXTERNAL DEFRIBILLATORS (AED)

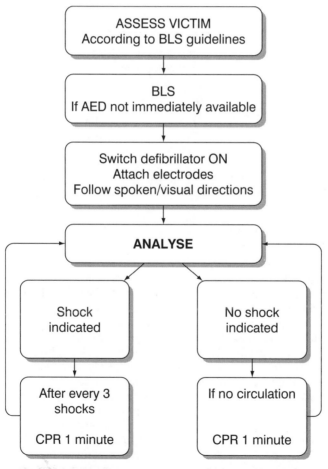

Continue until Advanced Life Support available

Redrawn with permission from the Resuscitation Council UK

ADVANCED LIFE SUPPORT ALGORITHM (ALS)

```
                        ┌─────────────────────┐
                        │   CARDIAC ARREST    │
                        └─────────────────────┘
                                  │
                        ┌─────────────────────┐
                        │ Follow BLS if appropriate │
                        └─────────────────────┘
                                  │
                        ┌─────────────────────┐
                        │ Precordial thump if appropriate │
                        └─────────────────────┘
                                  │
                        ┌─────────────────────┐
                        │ Attach defibrillator/monitor │
                        └─────────────────────┘
                                  │
                        ┌─────────────────────┐
                        │    Assess rhythm    │
                        └─────────────────────┘
                                  │
                        ┌─────────────────────┐
                        │    ±check pulse     │
                        └─────────────────────┘
```

| VF/VT | Non–VF/VT |

Defibrillate × 3 as necessary

CPR 1 min

CPR 3 min*
*1 min if immediately
after defibrillation

DURING CPR
Correct reversible causes if
  not already:
Check electrode/paddle
  positions and contact
Attempt/verify: airway and
  O₂ i.v. access
Give adrenaline/epinephrine
  every 3 minutes
Consider:
• Amiodarone
• Atropine/pacing
• Buffers

**Potentially reversible
  causes:**
Hypoxia
Hypovolaemia
Hyper/hypokalaemia and
  metabolic disorders
Hypothermia
Tension pneumothorax
Tamponade
Toxic/therapeutic disturbances
Thromboembolic/mechanical
  obstruction

CONSULT OTHER TOPIC

Deep vein thrombosis (p 248)

SUPPLEMENTARY INFORMATION

- Points 1–12 follow the Basic Life Support Guidelines of the European Resuscitation Council 2001.
- Point 16 follows the Advanced Life Support Guidelines.

Open airway by head tilt, chin lift and assess breathing for 10 seconds

Do this with the patient in the position in which you find her. Do this (but not if cervical spine injury is suspected), by

- Placing hand on the forehead and gently tilting head back keeping thumb and index finger free to close the patient's nose if rescue breathing is required.
- At the same time with your fingertips under the point of the patient's chin, lift the chin to open the airway. A jaw thrust may be required to open the airway. Do this by placing fingers behind the angle of the jaws and moving jaw anteriorly to displace tongue from the pharynx.
- If you have any difficulty turn the patient onto her back with a slight tilt to the left and then open the airway as described. Try to avoid head tilt if injury to the neck is suspected.

Give two rescue breaths

Do this by

- Ensuring head tilt and chin lift, pinching the soft part of the patient's nose closed with you thumb and index finger of the hand on the patient's forehead.
- Open her mouth a little but maintain chin lift.
- Take a breath and place your lips around her mouth, making sure that you have a good seal.
- Blow steadily into her mouth over 1.5–2 seconds watching for her chest to rise. The target tidal volume is 400–500 ml.
- Maintaining head tilt and chin lift take your mouth away from the patient and watch for her chest to fall as the air comes out.
- Take another breath and repeat the sequence as above to give another effective breath. If you have difficulty in achieving a breath recheck the patient's mouth for an obstruction, that head tilt and chin lift is adequate.

If circulation present but no breathing continue rescue breathing at a rate of 10 breaths/minute

Recheck the presence of circulation every 10 breaths taking no more than 10 seconds each time. If the victim starts to breath on her own but remains unconscious turn her into the recovery position and apply oxygen 15 l/minute. Check her condition and be ready to turn her back to restart rescue breathing if she stops breathing.

- If Automated External Defibrillator (AED) available, attach, analyse rhythm and defibrillate if indicated.
- The most frequent initial rhythm in cardiac arrest is ventricular fibrillation (VF). Successful defibrillation diminishes with time. The AED allows for early

defibrillation by lesser trained personnel as it performs rhythm analysis, gives information by voice or visual display and the delivery of the shock is then delivered manually.

- After first three shocks give uninterrupted CPR for 1 minute. If defibrillation is not indicated CPR should be continued for 3 minutes at which stage the AED will prompt further analysis of rhythm.

If no circulation (or you are at all unsure) start chest compressions after two initial breaths

With the patient tilted to the left locate the lower half of the sternum.

- Using your index and middle fingers identify the lower rib margins.
- Keeping your fingers together slide them up to the point where the ribs join the sternum. With your middle finger on this point place your index finger on the sternum.
- Slide the heel of your other hand down the sternum until it reaches your index finger; this should be the middle of the lower half of the sternum.
- Place the heel of one hand there, with the other hand on top of the first.
- Interlock the fingers of both hands and lift them to ensure that pressure is not applied over the patient's ribs. Do not apply any pressure over the top of the abdomen or bottom tip of the sternum.
- Position yourself above the patient's chest and with your arms straight press down on the sternum to depress it 4–5 cm.
- Release the pressure then repeat at a rate of about 100 times a minute. Compression and release should take an equal amount of time.
- To combine rescue breathing and compression after 15 compressions tilt the head, lift the chin and give two effective breaths.
- Return your hands immediately to the correct position and give 15 further compressions continuing this cycle of two breaths to 15 compressions.

Two person CPR is preferred if there are two rescuers. A ratio of five compressions to one ventilation should be used.

Attach defibrillator/monitor and assess cardiac rhythm

For defibrillation one paddle is placed to the right of the upper part of the sternum just below the clavicle, the other just outside the position of the normal cardiac apex, taking care to avoid breast tissue.

Turn immediately to ALS algorithm (p 236)

The majority of patients will have been successfully defibrillated in one of the first three defibrillating shocks. If the patient remains in VF a successful outcome relies on continued defibrillation and correction of causes or contributing factors.

If VF/VT can be positively excluded defibrillation is not indicated. The patient is in asystole or pulseless electrical activity (PEA). If PEA and HR < 60/min give atropine 3mg iv. The causes of cardiac arrest are hypovolaemia, total spinal anaesthetic or local anaesthetic toxicity, pneumo-thorax, cardiac tamponade, massive pulmonary embolus or amniotic fluid embolus or eclampsia.

Make decision to abandon CPR if unsuccessful

Do not abandon CPR if rhythm continues as VF/VT. Decision to abandon CPR should only be made after discussion with consultant obstetrician.

REFERENCE

The Resuscitation Council (UK) Guidelines for the use of Automated External Defibrillators.
In: *Resuscitation Guidelines 2000.* p 26.

ANAPHYLAXIS

Kate Grady

Anaphylaxis is an exaggerated response to a substance to which an individual has become sensitized in which histamine, serotonin and other vasoactive substances are released. This causes symptoms which can include pruritus, erythema, flushing, urticaria, angio-oedema, nausea, diarrhoea, vomiting, laryngeal oedema, bronchospasm, hypotension, cardiovascular collapse and death. Anaphylactic reactions usually begin within 5–10 minutes of exposure and the full reaction usually evolves within 30 minutes. Anaphylactic and anaphylactoid reactions are clinically indistinguishable and managed in the same way. They have a different immunological mechanism.

In a patient with latex allergy repeated vaginal examination with gloves containing latex and other exposure to latex can lead to anaphylaxis.

ACTION PLAN

1 **Diagnosis is made on clinical grounds – suspect**

2 **Stop administration of drug(s)/blood product likely to have caused anaphylaxis**

3 **Call for help including anaesthetist**

4 **Airway**
- Assess.
- Maintain patency.
- Apply oxygen 15 l/minute via tight fitting face mask with reservoir bag.
- Put on pulse oximeter.
- Consider tracheal intubation.

Breathing
- Assess.
- Ventilate.
- Protect airway.

Circulation
- Assess pulse, BP.
- CPR if necessary.
- Tilt to left.
- Put on ECG and BP monitor.
- Treat peri-arrest arrhythmias.
- Secure iv access with large bore cannula.

5 **Lie patient head down**

6 **Give adrenaline/epinephrine**
- Either 0.5–1 mg (0.5–1 ml of 1:1000) intramuscularly every 10 minutes until improvement in pulse and blood pressure.
  OR
- 50–100 μg (0.5–1 ml of 1:10 000) intravenously titrated against blood pressure.
- If cardiovascular collapse 0.5–1 mg (5–10 ml of 1:10 000) may be required intravenously in divided doses titrated against response. Give at a rate of 0.1 mg/minute and stop when a response has been obtained.

7   **Start intravascular volume expansion with crystalloid or synthetic colloid**

8   **Give secondary therapy**
- Antihistamines: chlorpheniramine 10–20 mg by slow iv infusion; consider ranitidine 50 mg iv.
- Corticosteroids: hydrocortisone 100–300 mg iv.

9   **Reassess airway, breathing and circulation**

10 **Consider catecholamines if blood pressure still low**
- Adrenaline/epinephrine 0.05–0.1 µg/kg/min (approx 4–8 µg/min). 5 mg adrenaline/epinephrine in 500 ml saline gives 10 µg/ml.
- Noradrenaline/norepinephrine 0.05–0.1 µg/kg/min (approx 4–8 µg/min); 4 mg noradrenaline/norepinephrine in 500 ml dextrose gives 8 µg/ml.

11 **Perform arterial blood gases**

12 **Consider bronchodilators if persistent bronchospasm**
- e.g. salbutamol 2.5 mg via oxygen driven nebulizer or 250 µg iv slowly. OR
- Aminophylline 250 mg iv over 20 minutes.

13 **Keep a record chart to include pulse, BP, RR, SaO$_2$ and treatments given**

14 **Document in notes with time, date, a signature and printed identification**

15 **Investigate**

CONSULT OTHER TOPIC

Acute severe asthma (p 259)

SUPPLEMENTARY INFORMATION

- Diagnosis is made on clinical grounds – suspect.
- The diagnosis is likely if flushing and urticaria, wheezing and hypotension coexist. Consider as a cause of cardiac arrest.

Clinical features	Frequency
Cardiovascular collapse	88%
Bronchospasm	36%
Angio-oedema	24%
(face, periorbital, perioral)	
Generalized oedema	7%
Cutaneous signs:	
Rash	13%
Erythema	45%
Urticaria	8.5%

First clinical feature	Frequency
No pulse, low BP	28%
Flushing	26%
Coughing	6%
Rash	4%
Cyanosis	3%
Others (urticaria, swelling)	9%

Stop administration of drug(s)/blood product likely to have caused anaphylaxis

As the cause, suspect any drug, infusion or blood or blood product currently being administered or given in the last 30 minutes. Anaphylactic reactions are more common when drugs are given intravenously.

Perform arterial blood gases

Sodium bicarbonate 8.4% should be given in increments of 50 ml where base excess is found to be –3 or acidosis is more severe. Blood gas analysis should be repeated between increments.

Document in notes

The doctor who administered/prescribed the drug/infusion/blood should ensure that the reaction is recorded appropriately in the notes. It is important to document timing of administration of all drugs in relation to onset of reaction. The responsible consultant should be informed immediately. The patient's GP must be notified. The patient should be given advice on further investigation, an explanation of events and a written record of the reaction. All suspected anaphylactic drug reactions should be reported to the Committee on the Safety of Medicines.

Investigate

Consider possibility of coagulopathy. Approximately 1 hour after the beginning of the reaction 10 ml of venous blood should be taken in a glass tube. The serum should be separated and stored at –20°C until it can be sent to a reference laboratory for serum tryptase concentration estimation which may be elevated in an anaphylactic reaction.

Any patient who has had a suspected anaphylactic reaction should be investigated fully. This is best done by referring the patient to an allergy clinic. The investigation should be conducted in consultation with an allergist or clinical immunologist. No blood test identifies the causative agent but other tests should be introduced on the advice of the allergist. Skin testing, radioallergosorbent testing (RAST) for specific drugs, or latex agglutination testing may be recommended. The British Society of Allergy and Immunology publishes a list of members able to advise.

Latex protein allergy

In care of these patients latex should be avoided therefore:

- Identify products containing latex and provide a list of alternatives.
- Ensure alternatives available and accessible at all times and kept in a specified place.

- Every member of staff having direct physical contact with the patient should ensure that whatever they wear or use does not contain latex.

The following products/equipment should not be used; latex containing gloves, Foley's in-dwelling catheters, iv sets with rubber injection site, Luer lock caps, rubber face masks, entonox rubber tubing, tourniquets, rubber mattress covers on theatre tables, beds, trolleys etc., sphygmomanometer tubing, elastoplast, multi dose bottles with rubber stopper e.g. lignocaine bottles.

REFERENCES

Ewan PW (1998) Anaphylaxis. *BMJ* **316**: 1442–1445.

The Association of Anaesthetists of Great Britain and Ireland and The British Society of Allergy and Clinical Immunology (1995) *Suspected Anaphylactic Reactions Associated with Anaesthesia.*

TRANSFUSION REACTIONS

Kate Grady

Allogenic blood transfusions (transfusion of blood from another individual) can result in transfusion reactions, anaphylactic or allergic responses or infection.

Acute transfusion reactions can be:

- Haemolytic.
- Non-haemolytic.

Haemolytic reactions can be:

- Intravascular (almost always due to transfusion of ABO incompatible blood).
- Extravascular (due to other antibodies).

ACTION PLAN

1 **During transfusion**
- Observe for first 15 min.
- Monitor temperature at 0, 15 and 30 min and then hourly from the start of each unit.
- Monitor pulse at 0, 15, and 30 min and then hourly.
- Monitor blood pressure at the beginning and half way through the unit (more frequently if other indication to do so).

2 **Suspect haemolytic transfusion reaction if pain in arms, loin or chest, dyspnoea, flushing or chills**

3 **Stop transfusion**
- Quickly check for ABO incompatibility. If ABO incompatible continue emergency management of symptoms. Alert blood bank immediately as blood intended for your patient could be transfused to another patient.

4 **Call for help including resident anaesthetist and inform haematologist**

5 **Airway**
- Assess.
- Maintain patency.
- Apply oxygen 15 l/min via tight fitting face mask with reservoir bag.
- Attach pulse oximeter to patient.

Breathing
- Assess.
- Ventilate.
- Protect airway.

Circulation
- Assess pulse and BP.
- CPR.
- Put on ECG monitor.
- Treat peri-arrest arrhythmias.
- iv access, send bloods for FBC, direct antiglobulin test (same tube), U&Es, LFTs, clotting studies, blood cultures and send 5 ml in dry tube for repeat compatibility testing.
- Treat hypotension.

6 **Consider anaphylaxis**

7 **Run normal saline 100–200 ml iv**

8 **Catheterize bladder and record urine output every 15 minutes**

9 **Give fluids to maintain urine output > 1.5 ml/kg/h**

10 **Consider need for CVP line**

11 **Give frusemide/furosemide 80–120 mg iv**
- If urine output < 1.5 ml/kg/hour and CVP > 0 cm H_2O and patient not hypotensive.

12 **Give mannitol 20% 100 ml if no diuresis after frusemide/furosemide**

13 **Assume acute renal failure and obtain specialist help**
- If 2 hours after frusemide/furosemide and mannitol urine output is < 1.5 ml/kg/h.

14 **Adjust infusion rate to maintain urine blood flow > 1.5 ml/kg/h**

15 **Call renal physicians if hyperkalaemic and check arterial blood gases to exclude acidosis**

16 **Repeat FBC, U&Es and coagulation screen 2–4 hourly. Send to blood bank remainder of blood unit and transfusion giving set**

17 **Contact consultant haematologist if coagulopathy**

18 **Contact consultant haematologist if patient needs further blood transfusion**

19 **Double check the labelling on the unit of blood with patient's identification band and with other identifiers**

20 **Late pyrexia or rigors in the absence of other signs are probably due to a non-haemolytic reaction**
- Stop transfusion, send sample and blood unit to blood bank and give aspirin 0.6–0.9 g po. Observe closely until symptoms and signs resolve. Discuss further transfusion with haematologist.

21 **Urticaria and itching at the start of transfusion in the absence of other signs are probably due to an allergic reaction**
- Give chlorpheniramine 4 mg po and stop transfusion for 30 minutes. If urticaria and itching resolve restart transfusion.

22 **For any reaction keep record chart of pulse, BP, RR, SaO$_2$, temperature and treatments given**

23 **Record reaction in notes chronologically with date, a signature, and printed identification and inform and explain to patient**

24 **Report serious adverse events following transfusion to Serious Hazards of Transfusion (SHOT) group**

CONSULT OTHER TOPICS

Anaphylaxis (p 240)
Cardiopulmonary resuscitation (p 234)

SUPPLEMENTARY INFORMATION

Suspect haemolytic transfusion reaction if pain in arms, loin or chest, dyspnoea, flushing or chills

Intravascular haemolytic reactions are rare but have a high mortality from disseminated intravascular coagulation (DIC) and acute renal failure (ARF).

They occur during the first few millilitres of transfusion and are characterized by pain in the arms, loin and chest, hypotension and red urine. Group A blood into a Group O patient causes the most severe reaction. Extravascular haemolytic reactions can cause an immediate, severe reaction if transfusion is rapid or a delayed reaction. Immediate severe reactions may lead to ARF.

Stop transfusion

Although haemolytic transfusion reaction is rare it can be fatal. Symptoms and signs appear after 5–10 ml. Prognosis is much worse if 200 ml or more have been given. Transfusion should be stopped as soon as a reaction is suspected.

Consider anaphylaxis

Very rarely severe anaphylaxis can occur (due to antibodies to IgA). Signs of anaphylaxis are angio-oedema, laryngeal oedema, bronchospasm, hypotension and cardiovascular collapse.

Run normal saline 100–200 ml iv

To maintain renal blood flow to prevent ARF. Hyperkalaemia and metabolic acidosis are signs of ARF.

Repeat FBC, U&Es and coagulation screen 2–4 hourly. Send to blood bank remainder of blood unit and transfusion giving set

Transfusion giving set is examined to exclude bacterial contamination as a cause of transfusion reaction.

Double check the labelling on the unit of blood with patient's identification band and with other identifiers

Direct antiglobulin test confirms a haemolytic reaction.

Late pyrexia or rigors in the absence of other signs are probably due to a non-haemolytic reaction

Non-haemolytic reactions are commonly called febrile reactions (due to white cell antibodies). They occur in approximately 1% of transfusions and are characterized by fever or rigors 30–60 min after the start of the transfusion.

Urticaria and itching at the start of transfusion in the absence of other signs are probably due to an allergic reaction

They are insignificant if there is no progression of symptoms after 30 min cessation of transfusion.

REFERENCE

Blood Transfusion Services of the United Kingdom (1996) *Handbook of Transfusion Medicine.*
 Her Majesty's Stationery Office, London

USEFUL TELEPHONE NUMBER

Serious Hazards of Transfusion (SHOT) Group   0161 273 7181

DEEP VEIN THROMBOSIS

Catherine Wykes and Kate Grady

Deep venous thrombosis (DVT) and pulmonary embolism (PE) are serious hazards in patients undergoing gynaecological surgery. They are a significant cause of post-operative morbidity and mortality. The reported incidence of DVT in patients undergoing gynaecological surgery ranges from 7 to 45% and fatal PE is estimated to occur in nearly 1% of these patients.

DEEP VEIN THROMBOSIS PROPHYLAXIS

ACTION PLAN

1 **Consider risk factors**

2 **Make a risk assessment of each patient**

3 **Assess medication pre-operatively and make any modifications required**

4 **Use subcutaneous heparin in all patients at high or moderate risk**

5 **Use anti-embolism stockings until fully mobile**

6 **Use peri-operative external pneumatic calf compression in high risk patients**

7 **Avoid dehydration in the post-operative period**

8 **Ensure early ambulation and encourage leg exercises**

9 **Consider continued prophylaxis following discharge in patients at high risk**

SUPPLEMENTARY INFORMATION

Consider risk factors

These risk factors apply to all forms of thromboembolic disease:

- Prolonged surgery (>30 minutes).
- Malignancy.
- Age >40 years.
- Prolonged immobilization.
- Obesity.
- Past history of PE or DVT.
- Varicose veins.
- Infection.
- Synthetic oestrogen therapy.
- Congenital and acquired thrombophilia.
- Smoking.
- Pregnancy.

Appendix 2

Make a risk assessment of each patient

Low risk

- Aged <40 years undergoing minor to intermediate surgery of less than 30 min duration.

High risk

- Aged >60 years undergoing major surgery.
- Aged >40 years with additional risk factors undergoing major surgery.
- Any patient undergoing major surgery with a past history of DVT or PE.

All other patients are at moderate risk.

Assess medication pre-operatively and make any modifications required

In the presence of other risk factors stop the COCP 4–6 weeks before major gynaecological surgery. Remember to discuss alternative methods of contraception.

There is no need to routinely stop HRT before surgery provided appropriate thromboprophylaxis is employed.

Subcutaneous heparin use in all patients at high or moderate risk

Give 5000 IU of low-dose unfractionated heparin subcutaneously 12 hourly if moderate risk or 8 hourly if high risk. The first dose is given 1–2 hours prior to surgery and continued 5–7 days post-operatively or until patient is fully mobile.

Low molecular weight (LMW) heparin (enoxaparin or dalteparin) are alternatives administered once daily. Give patients at moderate risk 20 mg/day or 2500 IU/day, respectively and those at high risk 40 mg/day or 5000 IU/day.

Use anti-embolism stockings until fully mobile

This is for all moderate and high-risk patients. In low-risk patient graded compression stockings and early ambulation are sufficient prophylaxis.

DEEP VEIN THROMBOSIS

ACTION PLAN

1 Have low index of suspicion for DVT

2 Identify risk factors for thromboembolic disease

3 Request Doppler

4 Do not delay starting treatment if index of suspicion is high and diagnostic tests cannot be performed rapidly

5 Take FBC, coagulation screen, U&Es, LFTs

6 Consult physicians

7 Start heparin, elevate leg and use graduated pressure stockings

8 Continue heparin until the diagnosis of DVT is excluded by objective tests

9 **If therapeutic anticoagulation with heparin is contra-indicated (e.g. due to high risk of bleeding) consider inferior vena cava filter**

10 **If large ilio-femoral thrombosis exists thrombolytic therapy or venous thrombectomy may be needed**

11 **Patients with objectively diagnosed DVT should receive anticoagulation for at least 3 months using warfarin or LMW heparin**

CONSULT OTHER TOPICS

Pulmonary embolism (p 252)

SUPPLEMENTARY INFORMATION

Have low index of suspicion for DVT

Clinical diagnosis of DVT is notoriously unreliable. Fifty to eighty percent of PEs occur without prior clinical evidence of DVT. In 10–20% of cases it is fatal.

Clinical features include calf pain, unilateral leg swelling with redness, engorged superficial veins and ankle oedema. The affected calf may be warmer.

Request Doppler

Venography is reliable but somewhat invasive. Duplex ultrasound imaging is as accurate as venography in femero-popliteal thrombosis but detects only 80% of calf-vein thrombosis. Venography is reserved for those who have a technically inadequate scan. Where doubt remains CT and MRI have a role.

Do not delay starting treatment if index of suspicion is high and diagnostic tests can not be performed rapidly

The main aim of treatment is to prevent PE. Prompt and adequate treatment is also important to reduce extension of DVT and hence morbidity from the post-thrombotic leg syndrome.

Take FBC, coagulation screen, U&Es, LFTs

This helps in the evaluation of risk factors for bleeding.

Start heparin, elevate leg and use graduated pressure stockings

Therapeutic doses of heparin, either unfractionated or LMW should be given either by iv or subcutaneous injection. LMW heparin is the treatment of choice as it can be given once daily and there is no need for routine monitoring of coagulation times and meta-analyses have shown greater efficacy, less risk of major bleeding and lower total mortality. Heparin should be continued until the diagnosis of DVT is excluded by objective tests.

Patients with objectively diagnosed DVT should receive anticoagulation for at least 3 months using warfarin or LMW heparin

When oral anticoagulant is initiated it should be overlapped with heparin therapy for 4–5 days until the INR is greater than 2 on 2 consecutive days. The optimum therapeutic range of the INR during oral anticoagulant therapy is 2.0–3.0. When oral anticoagulants are contraindicated or inconvenient, adjusted-dose subcutaneous unfractionated heparin therapy should be considered. LMW heparins are alternatives if warfarin is contraindicated.

PULMONARY EMBOLISM

Catherine Wykes and Kate Grady

Despite the proven benefits of mechanical and pharmacological modes of prophylaxis, PE remains a prevalent condition in surgical patients. It accounts for 3% of surgical inpatient deaths. Untreated clinically apparent PE has a 30% hospital mortality rate whereas mortality rates for treated patients have been reported at 2%. Early diagnosis and prompt effective management of this condition are vital.

1 **Remember risk factors**

2 **Suspect PE**

3 **Call senior gynaecologist and medical team**

4 **Perform basic resuscitation**
Airway
- Assess.
- Maintain patency.
- Apply oxygen 15 l/min via tight fitting face mask with reservoir bag.
- Attach pulse oximeter to patient.
- Consider early tracheal intubation if cardiovascular collapse or respiratory distress.

Breathing
- Assess.
- Ventilate with 100% oxygen if respiratory distress.
- May need positive end expiratory pressure to ventilate adequately.

Circulation
- Assess for signs of circulation and BP.
- CPR.
- Put on ECG and BP monitor.
- Secure large bore iv cannula, send FBC clotting studies and X-match, run IVI.
- If hypotensive give colloid.
- If massive PE consider central venous/pulmonary artery pressure monitoring.
- Manage hypotensive patients in ICU/HDU.

5 **Request CXR, ECG and ABGs**

6 **If high probability V/Q scan patient and anticoagulate**

7 **Pulmonary angiography, spiral computed tomography or MRI may be needed if V/Q scan is equivocal**

8 **Consider thrombolysis or pulmonary embolectomy if massive PE and patient is haemodynamically unstable**

9 **If positive diagnosis continue heparin anticoagulation and start warfarin**

SUPPLEMENTARY INFORMATION

Suspect PE

Clinical features are dyspnoea, tachypnoea, pleuritic pain, apprehension, tachycardia, cough, haemoptysis and clinical DVT with a descending order in frequency of 70–10%. Dyspnoea and a respiratory rate of >20 per minute occur in 90% of patients with acute PE; only 3% of patients have neither of these. Conditions presenting similarly include MI, pericarditis, pneumothorax and pneumonia.

Request CXR, ECG and ABGs

These are poor at diagnosing PE specifically but they may support the diagnosis. Importantly they help to exclude alternative diagnosis.

If high probability V/Q scan patient and anticoagulate

Give iv unfractionated heparin, 5000 IU bolus dose followed by maintenance intravenous infusion. Dosage should be adjusted to maintain APTT 1.5–2.5 control value.

A normal V/Q scan conclusively excludes a PE. If the result is unclear perform deep venous ultrasound to exclude DVT.

A normal D-dimer level, measured by ELISA, in patients with non-diagnostic V/Q scan excludes PE.

CONSULT OTHER TOPICS

Deep vein thrombosis (p248)
Cardiopulmonary resuscitation (p 234)
Myocardial infarction (p 254)
Chest infection (p 261)

MYOCARDIAL INFARCTION

Kate Grady and Ilan Lieberman

The emphasis is on early diagnosis and prompt management. Anaesthesia and surgery and illness may precipitate ischaemic heart disease and an increased risk of ischaemic heart disease and MI is present for several days post-operatively. Two percent of patients with ischaemic heart disease suffer a post-operative MI.

ACTION PLAN

1 **Airway**
- Assess.
- Maintain patency.
- Apply oxygen 15 l/min via tight fitting face mask with reservoir bag.
- Attach pulse oximeter to patient.

Breathing
- Assess.
- Ventilate.
- Protect airway.

Circulation
- Assess.
- CPR.
- Put on ECG and automatic NIBP monitor.
- Treat peri-arrest arrhythmias.
- iv access, send bloods for FBC, U&Es, blood glucose, cardiac enzymes CK, AST and LDH, G&S or X-match, start IVI. (Physician will advise on specific diagnostic test and timing.)
- Treat hypotension.

2 **Suspect**

3 **If history of ischaemic heart disease try sublingual glyceryl trinitrate**

4 **Call for senior physician or cardiologist**

5 **Get 12 lead ECG for diagnosis**

6 **Arrange CXR and arterial blood gases**

7 **Consider underlying cause and with physician treat expediently**

8 **Consider differential diagnosis**

9 **Arrange transfer to coronary care unit**

10 **Give analgesia – diamorphine 2.5–5 mg iv as required (with an antimetic cyclizine 50 mg iv)**

11 **With cardiologist consider anti-platlet therapy, aspirin 150 mg chewed**

12 **With cardiologist consider thrombolysis**

13 **Be aware of early complications**

14 **Keep record chart of pulse, BP, RR, SaO$_2$ and treatments given**

CONSULT OTHER TOPICS

Acute severe asthma (p 259)
Cardiopulmonary resuscitation (p 234)
Chest infection (p 261)
Peri-operative management of common pre-existing diseases (p 208)
Pulmonary oedema (p 257)
Pulmonary embolism (p 252)

SUPPLEMENTARY INFORMATION

Suspect

Suspect in the elderly and people with pre-existing ischaemic heart disease, valvular disease, hypertension, particularly if post-operative or systemically unwell.
  Presentation of an MI:

- Mild to severe central crushing chest pain at rest which may radiate to arms, jaw or upper abdomen.
- Restlessness.
- Grey and pallid.
- Sweating.
- Nausea.
- Vomiting.
- Hypotension.
- Breathlessness.
- Venous congestion crackles at lung bases.
- Pain may be silent especially in diabetics or hypertensives.
- May be pulmonary oedema.

A diagnosis of acute MI should be made if there is: Cardiac pain for at least 15 minutes, unrelieved by sublingual glyceryl trinitrate and ECG evidence of acute MI.

Get 12 lead ECG for diagnosis

ECG evidence of an MI includes at least 2 mm ST elevation in at least two contiguous pre-cordial leads, including right ventricular or lateral leads or at least 1 mm ST elevation in at least two inferior leads or leads 1 and aVL or left bundle branch block or signs of 'true posterior infarction', i.e. dominant R waves and deep ST segments in V1 and V2. If symptoms suggest acute MI but the ECG does not support the diagnosis, the ECG should be repeated once or twice at 15 minute intervals.

Consider underlying cause and with physician treat expediently

- Hypotension secondary to major haemorrhage.
- Illicit drugs (cocaine).
- Valvular rupture.
- Dissecting aortic aneurysm.

Consider differential diagnosis

- Anxiety.
- Heartburn.
- Pulmonary embolus.
- Pneumothorax.
- Pericarditis.
- Dissecting or enlarging aortic aneurysm.
- Valvular rupture.
- Pleurisy.
- Chest infection.
- Musculoskeletal pain.

Be aware of early complications

- Arrhythmias.
  Ventricular – life threatening.
  Sinus bradycardias and tachycardias.

PULMONARY OEDEMA

Kate Grady

Pulmonary oedema can present frankly with pink·frothy sputum or less floridly with breathlessness, tachycardia, cool peripheries, cyanosis and basal crepitations on chest examination.

The immediate diagnosis is usually obvious; what may be less obvious and is of importance in the management of the underlying cause.

ACTION PLAN

1 **Airway**
- Assess.
- Maintain patency.
- Apply oxygen 15 l/min via tight fitting face mask with reservoir bag.
- Attach pulse oximeter to patient.

Breathing
- Assess.
- Ventilate. IPPV is a treatment in itself for pulmonary oedema.
- Protect airway.

Circulation
- Assess.
- CPR.
- Put on ECG and automatic NIBP monitor.
- Treat peri-arrest arrhythmias.
- iv access, send bloods for FBC, U&Es, blood glucose, cardiac enzymes, CK, AST and LDH, G&S or X-match, start IVI.
- Treat hypotension.

2 **Call for senior anaesthetic and medical assistance**

3 **Sit upright if cardiovascularly stable**

4 **Consider underlying cause and simultaneously treat**

5 **Decrease preload with frusemide/furosemide 20–40 mg iv if cardiovascularly stable**

6 **Get 12 lead ECG, CXR and ABGs**

7 **In discussion with physician/anaesthetist decrease afterload with vasodilators (isosorbide, GTN)**

8 **In discussion with physician/anaesthetist decrease breathlessness with morphine 2 mg boluses iv to 10 mg**

9 **In discussion with anaesthetist consider IPPV**

10 **Transfer to high dependency/intensive care unit**

11 **Keep record chart of pulse, BP, RR, SaO$_2$ and treatments given**

CONSULT OTHER TOPICS

Cardiopulmonary resuscitation (p 234)
Myocardial infarction (p 254)

Appendix 2

Peri-operative management of common pre-existing diseases (p 208)
Pulmonary embolism (p 252)

Consider underlying cause and simultaneously treat

Increased pulmonary hydrostatic pressure

- Increased right atrial preload from fluid retention or fluid overload.
- Decreased myocardial contractility (MI or cardiomyopathy).
- Increased left atrial pressure (mitral stenosis).
- Increased afterload (hypertension, vasoconstriction).

Increased capillary permeability

- Adult respiratory distress syndrome (ARDS).
- Amniotic fluid, air or gas embolism.
- Pulmonary aspiration.
- Allergic reactions.
- Sepsis and pneumonia.

Other causes of pulmonary oedema

- Relief of obstructed upper airway.
- Neurogenic.

ACUTE SEVERE ASTHMA

Kate Grady

Asthma is caused by bronchospasm and is usually recognized by a wheeze.

Signs of severe asthma are being unable to complete sentences in one breath, RR > 25 breaths/min, HR greater than 110/min, use of accessory muscles of respiration and a peak expiratory flow (PEFR) of < 50% predicted (predicted = 480 l/min).

Signs of life threatening asthma are a silent chest, cyanosis or feeble respiratory effort, exhaustion, confusion, coma, bradycardia or hypotension and a PEFR of <33% predicted (approx 160 l/min).

PEFR can be measured at the bedside by asking the patient to exhale forcefully into a peak flow meter.

ACTION PLAN

1 **Call for help including resident anaesthetist, obstetrician and medical registrar**

2 **Give humidified oxygen 40–60%**

3 **Give salbutamol**
   - 5 mg in 3 ml normal saline as nebulizer via oxygen mask.

4 **Secure venous access, send bloods for FBC, U&Es, blood glucose and start iv fluids 1l normal saline/8 hourly**

5 **Give hydrocortisone 200 mg iv**

6 **Put on pulse oximeter**
   - If SaO_2 < 92% or patient has any life-threatening features measure arterial blood gases.

7 **Attach NIBP and ECG monitor**

8 **Check medical registrar has been summoned**

9 **Repeat PEFR measurement every 15 minutes**

10 **Repeat salbutamol 5 mg via nebulizer up to every 15 minutes until improvement**

11 **If life-threatening attack or not improving after 15 minutes**
   - Add ipratropium 500 µg to a repeat dose of salbutamol 5 mg via nebulizer.
   - Give iv aminophylline 250 µg over 10 minutes under ECG control, but not to patients already taking oral theophyllines

12 **Exclude tension pneumothorax; decompress if there is one**

13 **Be prepared to intubate and transfer to intensive care if respiratory arrest, deteriorating PEFR, persisting PaO_2 of < 8 kPa, deteriorating PaO_2, $PaCO_2$ of > 4 kPa, bradycardia, hypotension, exhaustion, confusion, coma or drowsiness – call anaesthetist**

14 **Organize portable CXR to exclude pneumothorax or consolidation**

15 **Send arterial blood gases**

16 **Consider cause of bronchospasm**

17 **Keep record chart of pulse, BP, RR, SaO_2 and drugs given**

18 **Record in notes and inform consultant**

CONSULT OTHER TOPICS

Cardiopulmonary resuscitation (p 234)
Anaphylaxis (p 240)

SUPPLEMENTARY INFORMATION

Give humidified oxygen 40–60%

CO_2 retention is not aggravated by oxygen therapy in asthma.

Give hydrocortisone 200 mg iv

Repeat 4 hourly if necessary.

Repeat PEFR measurement every 15 minutes

Improvement is signified by a rise in PEFR to above 50% predicted.

If life-threatening attack or not improving after 15 minutes

Add ipratropium 500 µg to a repeat dose of salbutamol 5 mg via nebulizer. Ipratropium may cause urinary retention.

Exclude tension pneumothorax

Signs of a tension pneumothorax include deviation of the trachea away from the affected side, reduced expansion of the chest on the affected side, hyperresonant percussion note on the affected side, reduced air entry on the affected side, tachycardia and hypotension.

The tension pneumothorax can be relieved in an emergency situation by inserting an intravenous cannula into the second intercostal space in the mid clavicular line on the affected side. A chest drain must be placed subsequently.

Send arterial blood gases

A $PaCO_2$ of > 4 kPa or a PaO_2 of < 8 kPa are signs of severe respiratory compromise.

REFERENCE

The British Thoracic Society *et al.* (1977) The British guidelines on asthma management 1995. Review and position statement. *Thorax* 1997; **52 (1):** S1–20.

CHEST INFECTION

Catherine Wykes and Kate Grady

The term 'chest infection' covers a wide variety of clinical presentations ranging from cough without sputum or chest signs to a more severe illness associated with mucopurulent sputum, fever, general malaise and dyspnoea.

Patients following surgery are at risk of developing chest infections for various reasons. They are at risk of atelectasis which may develop during general anaesthesia. Poor pain control post-operatively reduces deep breathing which compounds the process of atelectasis. Additionally patients who are not adequately starved pre-operatively may aspirate during anaesthesia. Pregnant patients are particularly at risk.

ACTION PLAN

1 **Take prophylactic measures**

2 **Remember risk factors for pulmonary atelectasis**

3 **Consider diagnosis**

4 **Perform U&Es, FBC (with differential WCC), blood cultures, CXR, sputum culture and microscopy**

5 **Sit the patient up**

6 **Maintain adequate hydration (iv fluids if necessary)**

7 **Refer for physiotherapy**

8 **Oxygen may be needed (but take care in COAD)**

9 **Start antibiotics**

10 **If the patient is very ill and does not respond to conventional treatment microbiological specimens may be obtained with the fibreoptic bronchoscope**

CONSULT OTHER TOPICS

Peri-operative management of common pre-existing disease (p 208)
Post-operative pain (p 230)

SUPPLEMENTARY INFORMATION

Take prophylactic measures

Liaise with anaesthetist/chest physician pre-operatively in patients with respiratory disease.

- Stop smoking pre-operatively.
- Do not perform elective surgery in patients with upper respiratory tract infection. Withhold surgery until at least 2 weeks after recovery.
- Ensure patient is adequately starved before surgery.
- Post-operatively start physiotherapy early and ensure analgesia is adequate.

Remember risk factors for pulmonary atelectasis

- Age.
- Obesity.
- Smoking.
- Poor post-operative analgesia.
- Upper abdominal incision.

Consider diagnosis

Patients may present with fever, pleuritic pain, cough, green sputum, haemoptysis and dyspnoea. Clinical signs include tachypnoea, unilateral dullness, pleural rub, bronchial breathing and crepitations.

Start antibiotics

If the patient is septic start iv therapy immediately. Antibiotic choice depends on the clinical picture. If the patient is very ill consult a microbiologist. In community acquired infection iv ampicillin (500 mg QDS) is usually the antibiotic of first choice converting to oral amoxycillin (250 mg TDS). This covers pneumococcus. Augmentin may be needed in haemophilus infections resistant to amoxycillin. If the patient gives a good history of allergy to penicillin or an 'atypical' infection is suspected give erythromycin. In hospital acquired infection give iv cefuroxime 750 mg TDS. In severe infections add iv gentamicin to cover gram-negative organisms. In cases of aspiration give iv cefuroxime, metronidazole and gentamicin.

PYREXIA OF UNKNOWN ORIGIN

Catherine Wykes and Kate Grady

Surgical patients are at risk of infection because post-operative organisms can gain entry to the tissues through an abnormal opening. Additionally physiological protective mechanisms may be disrupted e.g. increased risk of bronchopneumonia following anaesthesia and immobility and the patient's general resistance may be impaired by malnutrition, malignancy, steroid therapy or other immunosuppressive drugs.

The main pyogenic organisms of sugical importance are *Staphylococcus aureus*, some streptococci particularly *Streptococci pyogenes*, *Escherichia coli* and related gram-negative bacilli (coliforms) and bacteriodes. The use of prophylactic antibiotics dramatically reduces the incidence of post-operative abscess formation.

Common causes of early post-operative pyrexia (<36 h)

- Unexplained fever.
- Atelectasis.
- Urinoma.
- Ureteric obstruction.
- Wound infection.
- Transfusion reaction.
- Allergic drug reaction.

Common causes of late post-operative pyrexia (>36 h)

- Any of above.
- Urinary tract infection.
- Chest infection.
- Haematoma.
- Deep vein thrombosis.
- Pulmonary embolism.
- Septic thrombophlebitis.

ACTION PLAN

1 **Take a good history**

2 **Perform examination including vaginal examination if pelvic collection is suspected**

3 **Perform first-line investigations – FBC, ESR, U&Es, LFTs, blood culture (several from different veins), urinalysis, sputum for microscopy and CXR and wound swab**

4 **Second line investigations include ultrasound, CT, MRI, Doppler studies of leg veins and V/Q scan**

5 **Treat condition if suspected**

CONSULT OTHER TOPICS

Chest infection (p 261)
Pulmonary embolism (p 252)
Transfusion reactions (p 244)
Urinary tract infection (p 265)

SUPPLEMENTARY INFORMATION

Take a good history

The risk of atelectasis is increased by age, obesity, and history of smoking, inadequate post-operative analgesia and upper abdominal surgery. (Many patients with fever in the first 48 h do not have identifiable infection and the temperature settles without active treatment.)

Perform first-line investigations – FBC, ESR, U&Es, LFTs, blood culture (several from different veins), urinalysis, sputum for microscopy and CXR and wound swab

- An intermittent or spiking pyrexia suggests the presence of a loculated infection.
- In the presence of an abscess a full blood count reveals a marked neutrophil leucocytosis (WCC> 15 x 10 9/l) with more than 80% neutrophils.
- If patient has persisting diarrhoea send stool for microscopy.

Second line investigations include ultrasound, CT, MRI, Doppler studies of leg veins and V/Q scan

Ultrasound and CT scanning are valuable in abscesses. MRI is occasionally useful. Scanning with gallium-59 which is taken up by polymorphs or indium-111 labelled leucocytes can localize an abscess.

Other second line investigations include rheumatoid factor, ANA and Mantoux to exclude more rare causes such as connective tissue and autoimmune diseases and tuberculosis.

Treat condition if suspected

Condition	Treatment
Atelectasis	Physiotherapy and analgesia
Chest infection	Physiotherapy and amoxycillin
Urinary tract infection	Trimethoprim and fluids
Wound infection	Remove sutures, open wound, remove necrotic material, flucloxacillin or erythromycin if evidence of cellulitis
Septic thrombophlebitis	Remove cannula
DVT/PE	Anticoagulation
Faecal peritonitis	iv fluids and antibiotics, laparotomy
Ureteric obstruction	Percutaneous nephrostomy and ureteric stent or cystoscopy and retrograde ureteric stent
Urinoma	Refer urologist
Haematomas	Drain if fail to resolve spontaneously
Abscess	Incise and drain

URINARY TRACT INFECTION

Catherine Wykes and Kate Grady

UTI is common in women. Each year around 5% of women present with dysuria and frequency and about half have a UTI. UTI is more common in patients undergoing gynaecological surgery as the patient is usually catheterized pre-operatively. Increased risk is also associated with an in-dwelling catheter peri-operatively e.g. after uro-gynaecological surgery and radical vulvectomy.

If recurrent it may be a cause of considerable morbidity and can cause severe renal disease.

ACTION PLAN

1 **Remember risk factors**

2 **Consider prophylactic measures**

3 **Suspect UTI**

4 **Perform urine dipstick test**

5 **Obtain clean-catch midstream specimen of urine (MSU) and send for culture**

6 **If systemic signs of infection present take blood for FBC and blood culture**

7 **Encourage high fluid intake**

8 **Give analgesia or antipyretic for pain or fever**

9 **Start empirical treatment with antibiotics**

10 **If there is doubt that the infection has been eliminated repeat MSU 5 days after treatment**

11 **Refer to radiologist if patient develops recurrent, symptomatic and unexplained urinary infections**

SUPPLEMENTARY INFORMATION

Remember risk factors

- Female.
- Pregnancy.
- Urethral instrumentation.
- Renal stones.
- Conditions predisposing to urinary stasis.
- Co-existing pelvic disease e.g. tumours (may invade the bladder or alter its mechanical properties).
- Neurological disorders (may cause incomplete bladder emptying).
- Diabetes mellitus.

Consider prophylactic measures

If continuous bladder drainage is necessary post-operatively supra-pubic catheter should be used when appropriate. Consider antibiotics in patients at high risk.

Suspect UTI

Patients present with frequency, dysuria, suprapubic pain and tenderness, sensation of incomplete bladder emptying, haematuria and offensive urine. Acute pyelonephritis typically causes flank pain, nausea, vomiting, malaise or symptoms of cystitis.

Perform urine dipstick test

Tests for nitrites and/or leucocyte esterase (89% true positive and 66% true positive results, respectively).

Obtain clean-catch MSU and send for culture

More than 10^5 the same organism per millilitre indicates 'significant bacteriuria'. Lower bacterial counts can sometimes indicate clinically significant infections e.g. 10^2–10^4 ml^{-1} for symptomatic infections caused by gram-positive (e.g. *Staphylococcus saprophyticus*) or atypical organisms (e.g. proteus).

Most infections, are due to *E. coli* (70%), proteus mirabilis, klebsiella and *Staphylococcus saprophyticus*. In infections associated with anatomical, functional defects or iatrogenic causes, organisms isolated also include *Staphylococcus aureus*, coagulase-negative staphyloccoci and *Pseudomonas aeruginosa*.

Significant numbers of pus cells without bacterial growth are usually because patients are taking antibiotics. If not, a stone or tuberculosis must be suspected and investigated.

Start empirical treatment with antibiotics

Trimethoprim (200 mg twice daily), nitrofurantoin (50 mg four times daily) or oral cephalosporins are good first line drugs. Co-amoxiclav (375 mg three times daily) is an alternative for infections resistant to trimethoprim.

If the patient is acutely ill with acute pyelonephritis give iv cefotaxime (1 g twice daily) or an aminoglycoside (gentamicin 2–5 mg/kg daily in divided doses). While waiting for culture results. Switch to oral therapy as symptoms improve. Treatment should continue for 10–14 days.

If there is doubt that the infection has been eliminated repeat MSU 5 days after treatment

Also repeat in pregnant women, if the infection is complicated or in those with a history of recurrent infections.

Refer to radiologist if patient develops recurrent, symptomatic and unexplained urinary infections

Radiological imaging includes intravenous urography and ultrasonography to exclude anatomical abnormalities.

SEPTIC SHOCK

Kate Grady and Ilan Lieberman

DEFINITIONS

The term sepsis is often used inaccurately:

- *Sepsis* is defined as the presence of a systemic inflammatory response syndrome (SIRS) in conjunction with a demonstrated infection.
- *Severe sepsis* is defined as sepsis and organ failure.
- *Septic shock* is defined as sepsis and persistent hypotension despite adequate fluid resuscitation. It should be differentiated from other causes of shock.

ACTION PLAN

1 **Airway**
- Assess.
- Maintain patency.
- Apply oxygen 15 l/min via tight fitting face mask with reservoir bag.
- Attach pulse oximeter to patient.

Breathing
- Assess.
- Ventilate.
- Consider intubation if hypoxaemic.
- Protect airway.

Circulation
- Assess pulse, BP and note for bounding peripheral pulses and warm extremities.
- CPR.
- Put on ECG and automatic NIBP monitor.
- Treat peri-arrest arrhythmias.
- iv access, send bloods for FBC, U&Es, blood glucose, blood cultures, G&S or X-match, start IVI.
- Treat hypotension initially with volume replacement (inotropes will likely be required).

2 **Suspect**

3 **Call for anaesthetist and senior gynaecologist**

4 **Consider differential diagnosis of shock**

5 **Investigate to establish a focus of infection and treat obvious source**

6 **With advice of microbiologist start broad spectrum iv antibiotics**

7 **Consider transfer to high dependency unit/intensive care unit if appropriate and invasively monitor**

8 **Consider the use of inotropes**

9 **Monitor for and treat complications**

10 **Keep record to include pulse, BP, RR, SaO$_2$ and temperature**

CONSULT OTHER TOPICS

Anaphylaxis (p 240)
Cardiopulmonary resuscitation (p 234)
Chest infection (p 261)
Myocardial infarction (p 254)
Pyrexia of unknown origin (p 263)
Urinary tract infection (p 265)

Suspect

- Altered mental alertness.
- Vasodilatation bounding pulse and paradoxically warm periphery.
- Cyanosis.
- Tachycardia.
- Tachypnoea.
- Hypotension.
- Oliguria.
- Pyrexia.
- Nausea and vomiting.
- Multi-organ failure.
- Coagulopathy.

If hypotension does not respond to initial fluid bolus of 500 ml the diagnosis may be septic shock.

Consider differential diagnosis of shock

- Hypovolaemic.
- Obstructive.
- Cardiogenic.
- Histotoxic.
- Neurogenic.

Amongst many causes consider:

- Retained products.
- Unrelated other medical cause for sepsis – chest, urine, gut.
- Infected gestational sack.
- iv drug abuse.
- Iatrogenic – infected lines.
- HIV.

Investigate to establish a focus of infection and treat obvious source

Tests include blood cultures, urine microscopy and culture, throat, vaginal, wound swabs, CXR, FBC, differential white cell count, blood film and specific antibody titres.

Consider transfer to HDU/ICU if appropriate and invasively monitor

If the clinical picture of pyrexia, tachycardia, hyperdynamic peripheral circulation, wide pulse pressure and hypotension exists invasive monitoring of arterial, central venous and pulmonary artery pressures may be appropriate to optimize volume replacement and allow the use of inotropes.

Cardiovascular physiology is as follows:

- Low systemic vascular resistance (SVR).
- Low central venous pressure (CVP).
- Low pulmonary capillary wedge pressure (PCWP).
- High cardiac output (because of increased heart rate and stroke volume – stroke volume increased by ventricular dilatation).
- Later myocardial depression with low ejection fraction.

Monitor for and treat complications

The SIRS is defined by the presence of two of the following:

- Temperature >38 or < 36°C.
- Pulse >90.
- Respiratory rate >20 or pCO_2<32.
- WBC>12, <4, or > 10% band forms.

Acute renal failure, respiratory complications and DIC are recognized. Multi-organ dysfunction may develop.

CONFUSION

Kate Grady

Confusion is usually implied by irrational opinion or behaviour. It may be precipitated by anaesthesia and surgery or by illness. Attention must be paid to its cause.

ACTION PLAN

1 **Take history, examine and investigate to find cause and treat if applicable**

2 **If evidence of psychiatric illness take advice from psychiatrists**

3 **Give explanation and reassurance to patient**

4 **Consider issues of consent**

5 **Call consultant gynaecologist if there are issues of consent e.g. if surgery planned who will consider the best interest of the patient by balancing the need and risk. Consider telephone advice from his medical defence organization**

7 **Document, in full, decisions, to give treatment against patient's will or where treatment have been carried out without consent with time, date, a signature and printed identification**

8 **Retrospectively assess cause and follow up**

CONSULT OTHER TOPICS

Consent (p 279)
Risk management for medical staff (p 276)

SUPPLEMENTARY INFORMATION

Take history, examine and investigate to find cause. Treat if applicable

- Hypoxia.
- Hypotension.
- Sepsis.
- Drugs or drug withdrawal.
- Metabolic causes especially hypoglycaemia.
- Endocrine causes.
- Permanent mental disability.
- Psychiatric illness.
- Consider cerebral causes.

Consider involvement of neurologist if organic disease suspected.

If evidence of psychiatric illness take advice from psychiatrists

Improving the psychiatric illness may make the situation more manageable. Psychiatrist will consider whether a Treatment Order should be issued according to the Mental Health Act 1983. Note that even if the patient is sectioned under the Mental Health Act treatment can only be enforced for her psychiatric condition.

Give explanation and reassurance to patient

Try to address her anxieties. Attempt to 'talk down' aggressive patient and avoid confrontation.

Consider issues of consent

It must be decided whether the patient is capable of giving consent. This depends on her capacity to make an informed decision.

In the case of adults who are incapable of giving a valid consent, no parent, guardian or court has the power to consent on behalf of the patient. The issue of giving treatment to incompetent adults was addressed by the House of Lords in the case of F vs. West Berkshire Health Authority. The law lords confirmed that no one could consent on behalf of an incompetent adult but that it would be intolerable for adult incompetent patients to be denied treatment on the grounds that a consent could not be obtained. In these circumstances they said that doctors should act to protect the best interest of their patients by treating them in accordance with a responsible body of medical opinion.

If patients comply you may carry out investigation or treatment which you believe to be in their best interests. If they do not comply they can only be compulsorily treated for their mental disorder or a physical disorder arising from the mental disorder.

The 1983 Mental Health Act provides the legal basis for compulsory admission, detention and treatment.

REFERENCE

General Medical Council. Seeking patients' consent: the ethical considerations.

USEFUL TELEPHONE NUMBERS

Medical Defence Union	020 7935 5503
	0161 491 3301
Medical Protection Society	020 7399 1300
	0113 243 6436

Medical and Dental Defence Union of Scotland 0141 221 5858

EMERGENCIES IN TERMINAL ILLNESS

Kate Grady, Kim Hinshaw and Charles Cox

With adequate pre-operative investigation, good imaging techniques and appropriate and timely referrals it is to be expected that the gynaecologist would encounter very few emergencies of terminal illness. This chapter is included however to ensure awareness and good management in the exceptional circumstance.

However, some patients with terminal disease are given 'open access' to gynaecological services for the management of their gynaecological/urinary symptoms.

Advice can be taken from hospital palliative care teams, community palliative care nurses and hospice staff.

Terminal symptoms occur in approximately these percentages of patients in the last 48 hours of life:

Respiratory distress	56%
Pain	50%
Agitation	40%
Incontinence of urine	30%
Urinary retention	20%
Nausea and vomiting	14%

RESPIRATORY DISTRESS

ACTION PLAN

1 Put on pulse oximeter and if saturation is < 92% give oxygen via face mask with reservoir bag at 10–15 l/minute. If history of pulmonary disease with CO_2 retention give 24% oxygen

2 Sit upright

3 Reassure and calm patient

4 Increase air movement over patient's face

5 If stridor (i.e. obstructive noise on inspiration) is present call an anaesthetist

6 Consider pulmonary oedema as a cause

7 Consider pain in thoracic area as a cause (see pain section in this chapter)

8 Consider pulmonary embolism as a cause

9 Give hyoscine 20 mg sc if retained secretions

10 Consider oramorph 2.5–20 mg 4 hourly

11 Consider nebulized morphine 5–10 mg in 5 ml saline 2–4 hourly

12 Call palliative care team

CONSULT OTHER TOPICS

Pulmonary embolism (p 252)
Pulmonary oedema (p 257)

PAIN

1 Take a detailed history

2 Be aware there may be a number of pains

3 If pain is severe and overwhelming give diamorphine 5 mg iv, sc or im if not on strong opioid or half of the usual 4 hourly oral dose or one twelfth of the total 24 hourly oral intake by one of these routes and call palliative care team urgently. Consider fentanyl lozenge if on strong opioid already (200 µg lozenge)

4 For less severe pain start codeine 30–60 mg 4 hourly. If pain uncontrolled by this start morphine 5–10 mg 4 hourly orally and prescribe same oral dose 2 hourly for breakthrough pain

5 Start an NSAID (ibuprofen 800 mg TDS) or COXIB (celecoxib 200 mg BD) unless contraindicated

6 Consider neuropathic pain and consider starting amitriptyline or nortryptyline 10–25 mg ON

7 Call palliative care team

AGITATION

1 Assess cause e.g. hypoxia, dehydration, drugs or drug withdrawal, infection, biochemical derangement

2 Address cognitions, offer support, counselling and ensure safe environment

3 Consider lorazepam 0.5–1.0 mg orally or sublingually or midazolam 1 mg increments iv (call anaesthetist if doing this as respiratory depression can occur), or haloperidol 5–10 mg im if there is an element of psychosis

4 Call palliative care team urgently

INCONTINENCE OF URINE

1 Exclude infection

2 Exclude overflow incontinence (e.g. pelvic mass/faecal impaction)

3 Consider detrusor instability/neurogenic bladder (check sensation in 'saddle' area)

4 Improve mobility and access to toileting facilities

5 Consider bladder specific anticholinergic if indicated

6 Use formal 'bladder drill' if indicated (i.e. gradual increase in voiding interval)

7 Ensure appropriate nursing care to vulval/perineal skin and pressure areas

8 Involve specialist incontinence advisor

9 Provide incontinence aids

10 Catheterize – should be last manoeuvre in action plan

URINARY RETENTION

ACTION PLAN

1 Treat overt urinary tract infection with appropriate antibiotics

2 Treat 'reversible' causes (e.g. faecal impaction) and consider 'irreversible' causes (e.g. inoperable pelvic mass)

3 Catheterize (aseptic technique)

4 Use gel as urethral lubricant (consider local anaesthetic gel)

5 Use 12–14F Foley catheter

6 Only 10 ml is required in retaining balloon (using more will not prevent catheter by-passing)

7 Use *silastic* type Foley catheter if planning to leave catheter >10 days

8 If long-term catheterization – train patient in use of leg-bag

9 If long-term catheterization – consider insertion of supra-pubic catheter

10 Treatment of +ve CSU is not indicated in *asymptomatic* patients

11 There is no benefit in 4 hourly clamping/release to try and maintain bladder tone

12 Involve specialist incontinence advisor

FISTULAE PRESENT DISTRESSING PROBLEMS TO THE PATIENT, RELATIVES AND CARERS

- Vesico-colic fistulae cause frequency, dysuria and painful bladder spasm because of infection.
- A recto-vaginal fistula causes faecal incontinence and discharge and consideration should be given to a defunctioning colostomy.
- Urinary incontinence from a small vesico-vaginal fistula can be helped by vaginal tampons.
- Larger fistulae may be managed by a urinary catheter placed in the vagina inside a vaginal prosthesis.
- Urine output at night can be reduced by the use of desmopressin.

NAUSEA AND VOMITING

ACTION PLAN

1 Consider cause and treat as appropriate e.g. dehydration, drugs, obstruction, hypercalcaemia or raised intracranial pressure

2 Remember established nausea is associated with gastric stasis so oral antiemetics are ineffective – oral antiemetics are used to prevent nausea e.g. prochlorperazine 5 mg TDS or haloperidol 1.5 mg ON

3 To treat an episode of nausea use prochlorperazine 12.5 mg im or cyclizine 50 mg im

4 For established nausea use prochlorperazine 50 mg PR TDS or cyclizine 50 mg PR TDS or chlorpromazine 100 mg PR ON

5 Subcutaneous infusions of antiemetics may be necessary e.g. cyclizine 150 mg/24 h

6 Twenty-five percent of those suffering from nausea and vomiting need two antiemetics. Ondansetron may be necessary – take advice from palliative care team

FURTHER READING

Blackledge, Jordan and Shingleton (1991) *Textbook of Gynaecologic Oncology*. W.B. Saunders.

Appendix 2

APPENDIX 3

RISK MANAGEMENT FOR MEDICAL STAFF

Charles Cox and Kate Grady

Risk management is essential for safe gynaecological practice. Litigation against Trust doctors and nurses has increased dramatically as have complaints about all aspects of medical care. Medical staff of all grades should belong to a medical defence organization. Many cases are now settled on a no blame basis to avoid the cost of going to court even with cases which at first sight seem eminently defensible.

1 ALWAYS obtain consent or confirmation of consent before carrying out a procedure. The consent should be informed and the patient capable of understanding. It is the surgeon's responsibility. If possible give the patient an appropriate information leaflet especially for procedures such as sterilization where failure rates and complications need to be clearly stated. Record in the notes and the letter from the clinic what you have told the patient and if you have any concerns write a letter to the patient to reinforce the consultation. Consent should be witnessed and if necessary the consent can be countersigned. Get an interpreter if needed. Draw diagrams and leave them in the notes

2 ALWAYS have a chaperone present for examinations – it does not matter which sex you are! Explain to the patient what you are about to do. Even listening to a patient's chest, examining their legs or palpating their abdomen may be open to misinterpretation. However, the patient should always have the opportunity to speak to you in private before and after the examination

3 ALWAYS keep clear records which are timed, dated and signed with your name printed underneath. Many hospitals now issue stamps with the doctor's name and GMC registration number. As part of auditing risk management some departments do random checks on notes to check that this information is being entered into the notes and take disciplinary action against staff who do not comply. Remember good notes equals good defence, poor notes equals poor defence and no notes equals no defence

4 ALWAYS record clearly drug prescriptions, iv infusion prescriptions and allergies

5 ALWAYS be meticulous in writing up operative notes. With the availability of video equipment and digital or polaroid cameras it will often be helpful to have a visual record of operative findings for example in the case of failed sterilization. In a case of failed sterilization make sure there is another senior member of medical staff available to witness the findings at further laparoscopy or laparotomy

6 ALWAYS be honest – difficulties often occur in surgery. The test is how you deal with them. Be unafraid to ask colleagues from your

own or other specialties for advice and assistance. This is not a sign of inadequacy rather the reverse! Clearly describe the complication and the procedure used to deal with it and other people involved

7 ALWAYS inform a senior clinician if there has been a problem and make sure that the patient is informed of any complication likely to affect the speed of their recovery or the success of the operation

8 ALWAYS, if you suspect that an incident may become the subject of a complaint, obtain contemporaneous statements from witnesses and discuss them with the consultant gynaecologist and the clinical risk manager. Have a high index of suspicion. If you suspect a potentially litigious situation is developing record the events but do not place this record in the notes. Keep a copy yourself and forward one to your risk manager

9 ALWAYS record patient refusal to comply with suggested treatment and have it witnessed

10 ALWAYS tell the truth

11 NEVER ever alter the records. Even if grossly inaccurate or libellous. Write a revised version with timings, dates and signature with printed name and GMC registration number underneath

12 NEVER under any circumstances erase or delete any part of the record. This includes reports of scans, blood results and correspondence

13 NEVER criticize a colleague in front of a patient or the patient's relatives and never enter criticisms into the notes. For that matter it is best not to criticize any member of the medical or nursing team in public. If concerned about a colleague's performance discuss this with the clinical/medical director or if you are a junior member of staff with your educational supervisor/district tutor or the senior member of the junior staff. It is our responsibility to report concerns and we will be open to justified criticism if we do not

14 NEVER record any personal remarks or derogatory comments about the patient or her relatives in the notes. However, records should be kept in the notes of aggressive behaviour, bad language, threats and evidence of intoxication or substance abuse

15 NEVER delegate inappropriately and when delegating make sure that the individual knows exactly what is to be done and where senior cover can be found

CONSULT OTHER TOPIC

Consent (p 279)

SUPPLEMENTARY INFORMATION

There has been a rapid increase in legal actions relating to gynaecological procedures particularly to do with sterilization and termination of pregnancy. The reasons for this include increasing but often unrealistic expectations of what can be achieved. This has been encouraged by government and paradoxically by many Trusts.

Many problems arise from poor communication both with the patient, the patient's relatives and advocates and between members of the medical and nursing staff. This is increasing because of the loss of continuity arising from the loss of the team system. Formal handovers are becoming as important in gynaecology as in obstetrics.

- Inadequate supervision leads to litigation.
- Fear of litigation paradoxically often leads to worse care.
- Doctors may not be able to rely on their employers to look after their interests and should therefore retain membership of a medical defence organization.

USEFUL TELEPHONE NUMBERS

Medical Defence Union	020 7935 5503
	0161 491 3301
Medical Protection Society	020 7399 1300
	0113 243 6436
Medical and Dental Defence Union of Scotland	0141 221 5858

CONSENT

Keith Allenby, Kate Grady and Charles Cox

Informed consent means that the patient has all the necessary information to make a decision regarding their submission to a procedure. It is defined as 'a voluntary uncoerced decision, made by a sufficiently competent or autonomous person, on the basis of adequate information and deliberation, to accept rather than reject some proposed course of action that will affect her.'

The competent adult has a right under law to withhold consent to examination, investigation or treatment and to treat, investigate or have physical contact without consent may amount to assault.

CONSENT IN ANY SETTING

- Consent may be implied by the conduct of the patient in co-operating e.g. to examination. Any procedure which carries a material risk should carry express consent which may be oral or written.
- It is the responsibility of the doctor taking consent to ensure the patient is willing, has the ability to understand what is involved and has sufficient information (of potential outcome and risk) to make a judgement. The patient must understand the need for the operation, the expected outcome of the operation, the risks and their physical state post-operatively e.g. catheters, packs, drips, drains etc. If it is thought that a stoma is likely this should be fully discussed and a stoma nurse visit the patient prior to surgery. The effect of the operation on sexual function should be discussed. If the ovaries are to be removed hormone replacement therapy should be discussed. It should be clear to the patient who is likely to be doing the operation.
- Ensure an adequate interpreter; sensitivity should be given to this e.g. a young son should not be asked to interpret for a discussion about sexual dysfunction.
- Operations where one should be especially careful with regard to consent are sterilization, termination of pregnancy, removal of the ovaries when it is at the surgeon's discretion and the formation of a stoma.
- If you are not able to fully discuss failure and complication rates you must consult more senior staff.
- If in doubt that the patient has fully understood or in cases where the consent is complicated, write a letter to the patient with a copy to the GP.
- It should be the normal practice for the surgeon who is to carry out the operation to obtain consent. He or she should also be present when the consent form is signed. In practice this may be difficult. If consent has been obtained in outpatients, it is advisable for the operating surgeon to go over the proposed operation again to ensure the patient fully understands the need for the operation and the expected outcome of the operation.
- Written information leaflets explaining outcome and risk are useful supplements to discussion with a later opportunity to discuss their content. A record of the patient having been given the written information should be made in the notes.
- Risk is one which would be defined by a reasonable body of medical opinion as having significance or one which would have significance for the patient e.g. the risk of loss of sight in one eye becomes significant if you have sight in one eye only to start with.
- A contemporaneous record of the discussion surrounding informed consent should be made in the notes. In some cases it is sensible to have a witness and

for that witness to sign the consent form. This will often be the nurse from the ward or clinic.

- A consent form is a record of willingness alone. It is not a legal requirement.
- If consent has not been given and emergency treatment is required a consultant should take the decision. In doing so a consultant should discuss the case with a consultant colleague and document the discussion.

CONSENT FOR MINORS

- The United Nations Convention on Rights of the Child and the Children Act 1989 establish the child's right to be consulted.
- The Gillick principle states that 'the child's full consent is required if the child is of sufficient understanding to make an informed decision', which is for the doctor to decide. It has established a precedent for treating a child without parental consent if the child is judged competent. This may be applied to young women under 16 requesting abortion without parental knowledge.
- The above is open to interpretation and makes no distinction between the giving and refusing of consent and tacitly acknowledges that children mature at different rates.
- Children can only truly consent if they understand the nature, purpose and hazards of the treatment.
- In most cases, consent should be confirmed with the child's parent or guardian.
- Jehovah's Witnesses – for children under the age of 16 without capacity to consent the doctor's duty is to the patient and he or she may give blood or blood products if they are a necessary component of the relevant treatment, regardless of parental wishes. (High Court permission may be needed.)
- A parental refusal of advance consent to an operation considered necessary to the child's health may be challenged in the High Court.

CONSENT IN MENTAL ILLNESS OR LEARNING DIFFICULTY

- Being competent means having the ability to comprehend and retain information, believing the information and being able to use the information to make a decision.
- The mentally ill patient or the patient with learning difficulty must be able to understand what the treatment is, why it is being suggested, the consequences of not having treatment and must be able to retain the information for long enough to make a decision.
- If there is doubt about this take advice from a psychiatrist.
- Record your assessment of mental capacity in the notes.
- The hospital legal advisor should be consulted and a decision taken whether the woman has mental capacity and whether an application should be made to the courts to detain the woman under The Mental Health Act 1983.

CONSULT OTHER TOPICS

Peri-operative management of patient declining blood and blood products (p 227)
Risk management for medical staff (p 276)
Therapeutic abortion – indications and the Abortion Act (p 87)

REFERENCES

General Medical Council. Seeking patients' consent: the ethical considerations
Panting GP (1998) *Consent*. Prepared for members of the Medical Protection Society.

USEFUL TELEPHONE NUMBER

General Medical Council   020 7580 7642

INDEX